NORTH IDA

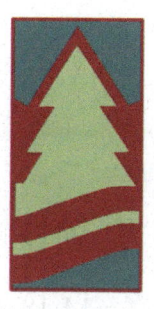

Published By: Kendall Direct Publishing

Copyright @2020 by: Doug Eastwood

This book is a non-fiction, historical account of the North Idaho Centennial Trail. The information contained within the book was gathered from archives of public agencies, newspapers, libraries, North Idaho Museum, and from trail supporters that kept their own historical records of this phenomenal project.
All rights reserved. No part of this book may be reproduced, scanned, or distributed in any printed, electric or audio form without written permission. All proceeds from the sales of this book will go to the North Idaho Centennial Trail Foundation.

ISBN – 9798535193144

PRINTED IN THE UNITED STATES OF AMERICA

First Edition – February 2020

Second Edition – August 2021

THE TRAIL THAT ALMOST WASN'T

Table of Contents

Prologue		4-5
Chapter 1	Getting Started With A Route Through History	6-13
Chapter 2	A Movement	14-18
Chapter 3	Benefits of the Trail	19-26
Chapter 4	The Bridge	27-39
Chapter 5	The Cost of Building a Trail	40-45
Chapter 6	Corbin Ditch	46-49
Chapter 7	Trouble in the Hood	50-56
Chapter 8	The Fight Over Old Highway 10	57-63
Chapter 9	Federal Appropriation Halted	64-67
Chapter 10	The Death of the Trail	68-69
Chapter 11	The Lumber Mills	70-75
Chapter 12	Where There is Smoke...	76-79
Chapter 13	A Disconnected Trail	80-82
Chapter 14	Seltice Way and Interstate 90	83-84
Chapter 15	Slip Slidin' Away...	86-92

Chapter 16	Long-Term Problem Solving	93-99
Chapter 17	Rails to Trails	100-103
Chapter 18	Naming a Premier Idaho Trail	104-105
Chapter 19	Millennium Legacy Trail	106-108
Chapter 20	North Idaho Centennial Trail Foundation	109-111
Chapter 21	Twenty-Three Stories	112-169
Epilogue		170-172
Points of Interest		173-197
References & Notes		198-200
Acknowledgments		201
About the Author		202-203

The North Idaho Centennial Trail

The Trail That Almost Wasn't

Prologue

The freedom of running and bicycling along the Centennial Trail has become a common experience. Feeling the breeze of the air as you travel along the trail corridor taking in the sights and sounds. Watching the water spill over the dam and mesmerizing dance of the sun light and moon light as they play upon the lake and the river. These are just a few of the things that we enjoy when we engage with the Centennial Trail.

Imagine that the North Idaho Centennial Trail does not exist. It does not cross the Spokane River on a historic railroad bridge. There is no trail connectivity between the City of Post Falls and the City of Coeur d'Alene. It does not meander through our community providing access to parks, neighborhoods, schools and scenic viewpoints. Suppose that you as a trail user could never experience the views of the Spokane River and Lake Coeur d'Alene while celebrating the Centennial Trail.

It is nothing short of a miracle that the Centennial Trail exists today. The size and cost of this project was the first of its kind in Kootenai County. Fear was raised by residents that the trail would lower property values, increase crime, and be dangerous for children. Political differences further divided the community on how our public roadways should be used, and who should be allowed to access them. There were times when it was thought that the trail would not come to fruition, and the idea of this trail in our community should be abandoned.

The concept of a trail began in late 1986, and while the North Idaho Centennial Trail has been enjoyed by millions of people for the last 30 years, the development of the trail did not come easy. The trail project had been stalled on numerous occasions. Thirty years have passed since the ground breaking of the first five miles of the trail in 1990. Trail users and enthusiasts expressed a need to capture in writing the history and sometimes tumultuous story of this 23-mile linear park system. Every life enriched by the Centennial Trail will have a greater appreciation for this lasting legacy when they read how, against all odds, this magnificent trail came to be.

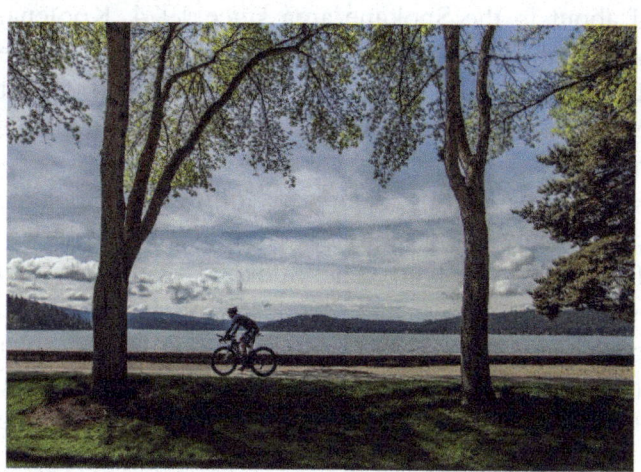

Photo by Jon Jonkers

Chapter 1
Getting Started With A Route Through History

A pedestrian and bicycle trail had been talked about as early as 1974 during the World's Fair held in Spokane, Washington that year. The fair organizers had envisioned a trail system to connect Spokane with the Washington/Idaho state line. Nearly 12 years later that vision was being resurrected. Washington, and Idaho, were approaching their respective states centennials; 1989 and 1990. The trail idea was being expanded to connect Spokane all the way to Coeur d'Alene, ID.

In 1986, a meeting was held in Spokane, Washington for the purpose of discussing the trail idea that had been talked about in the Spokane area since 1974. Kootenai County Commissioner Evalyn Adams, Coeur d'Alene City Council member Bob Mcdonald, and myself, Coeur d'Alene Parks Director Doug Eastwood, attended this first meeting.

There was a strong desire to follow the Spokane River as closely as possible and recapture the historical significance of the land. The Spokane, Kalispell, and Coeur d'Alene tribes had been in this area for an estimated 7,500 years. They would canoe on the river and fish the abundant supply of salmon. The natives traveled on foot from village to village, establishing well-worn trails along the river.

"The river was central to the Indian community. All along the river, there are significant historical sites that should be emphasized," Robert Dellwo, a Spokane City Councilman at that time shared. The excitement that stemmed from that initial meeting was contagious.

City Councilman Bob Mcdonald, introduced to Coeur d'Alene the idea of a bi-state trail that would connect Spokane to Coeur d'Alene. Bob wanted to form an exploratory committee to examine the feasibility of developing such a trail system in Idaho. The city council endorsed Bob's idea unanimously. He further informed the city council that he would like to have the city parks director, me, appointed to chair the exploratory committee. I saw this as a daunting task and realized it would take a lot of dedicated people, if not a community, to accomplish such a project.

Bob Mcdonald and Evalyn Adams became members of the exploratory committee. Bob rode a bike for recreation around his neighborhood and in the downtown area. Evalyn would walk her dog frequently around Tubbs Hill. I was a long-distance bicyclist. All three of us recognized a need for safe trail corridors that could also be used for commuting to work or to points of interest. We had a passion to see this idea come to fruition. Someone from the running community was needed to be on this exploratory committee. Runners, like bicyclists and walkers, did not have a safe place to run.

I reached out to Randy Haddock and Gary Bartoo, two names that are synonymous with running. They were both involved with the North Idaho Road Runners who started the Coeur d'Alene Marathon, which is now into its 40th year. I met with, and explained, to them the bi-state trail idea. Both Randy and Gary were interested and wanted to know how much time might be required to see this project come to fruition. They were told it might take anywhere from one to three years to complete the project. Randy agreed to join the exploratory committee, which quickly became the trail committee. Gary offered to assist wherever he might be needed but could not commit to joining the group at that time as he was establishing a physical therapy business.

The City of Post Falls city council was presented with the idea, and they too embraced the concept. City Councilwoman Karen Streeter and Parks Director Lance Bridges, became members of the trail committee representing Post Falls. The trail committee began meeting regularly in January of 1987. We met bi-weekly at the city owned Jewett House at the east end of East Lakeshore Drive. Individuals interested in this trail idea were invited to attend. The bi-monthly meetings were averaging 20 people in attendance; all were excited and passionate about the trail concept.

City maps were studied to identify potential routing of the trail from the state line to Coeur d'Alene. The idea appeared to be possible but it was time to hire a firm to do an in-depth review of routing and estimates of probable costs to build the trail.

The cities of Post Falls and Coeur d'Alene jointly financed a trail master plan. A land planner was hired in 1987 to identify the trail route and provide estimates of cost to construct the trail. Architects West/Landmark landed the assignment, with Landscape Architect, Jon Mueller, the lead person on the project. Historical sites along the trail corridor were identified by the Landscape Architect, this was like a step back in time for him while planning a viable route.

Planning a trail route over a 23-mile corridor required the identification of public and private land. Public land could be on roadways that would have enough right-of-way to include a trail. Public land could also provide access through parks, or land owned by a municipality, other than a park or a street. Private land could be property adjacent to a public street that could be used to expand the street to accommodate a pedestrian trail. It could also include land held by corporations such as a railroad. Public land usually meant access to that property without cost other than trail construction costs. Private land could lead to purchasing the needed property and escalating the cost of the trail development.

There are three classes of trails that were used during the planning stages. Class I would be a trail that is physically separated from vehicle traffic. This is the safest and preferred class of trail. However, developing a class I trail along the entire route would prove to not be feasible.

Class II trails have a designated pedestrian/bicycle lane but are usually immediately adjacent to vehicle traffic. This class of trail is usually found on public roadways and it is preferable to have a designated class II trail on both sides of the road. The designated pedestrian lane is most often identified with a painted stripe that is wider than typical vehicle lane striping. This painted line is also referred to as a 'fog' line.

Class III trails share the road with vehicle traffic. This class of trail identifies the route, but pedestrian and vehicles travel on the same roadway without any physical separation, or painted lines. Vehicles and pedestrians are mixed together. Bicycle etiquette is that of following the same rules as those applied to vehicles. Bicycles should travel in the same direction as vehicle traffic and stay as far to the right as possible. Those rules do not apply to runners as they prefer to run in the opposite direction of vehicle traffic. For them, class I is the preferred type of trail, and class III is the least preferred.

The task of identifying the route and trail classes fell to the Landscape Architect and included considerable interaction with the trail committee.

THE TRAIL THAT ALMOST WASN'T

Crossing the Spokane River became the first hurdle to making the bi-state connection. Fortunately, Burlington Northern Santa Fe Rail Road (BNSF) had abandoned their railroad bridge in 1974 and the trail committee thought that would be the perfect connection. Unfortunately, BNSF had just entered into an agreement with Acme Concrete of Spokane. Acme Concrete wanted to buy the bridge for their own transportation needs. This would pose a *huge* problem for the trail project.

BNSF was also abandoning some of their right of way from Pleasant View Road to Spokane Street in Post Falls. Trail planners looked at that property to connect the trail from the state line into the City of Post Falls. BNSF did not have a pending sale on this property yet, so a letter of interest was sent to them. They responded with a $139,000 price tag for the nearly three-mile corridor. It was great that the property was available. The difficulty in making the purchase is that there were no available funds.

The Corbin Irrigation Canal had also been abandoned nearly 50 years earlier. The canal, also referred to as the 'Corbin Ditch,' was constructed by Daniel Corbin in the late 1800's to bring water into the Spokane Valley for agriculture. Not wide enough to accommodate both bicycles and pedestrians, the ditch could serve as a nice pedestrian trail with a bicycle trail along side of it. When the idea of using the Corbin Ditch as a trail was shared at the first public meeting, concerns were raised from adjoining property owners about possible trespassing, litter, and dog waste.

Lumber was a major economic engine in the region at that time, with eight lumber mills on or near the proposed route. The lumber mills also opposed the trail route with vigor in the upcoming years. The mills successfully lobbied the Post Falls Highway District, who had jurisdiction over part of the recommended route. They, in turn, would take a position of denying trail access to the public roads. The Post Falls Highway District threatened law suits prohibiting trail use of their jurisdictional roads if the trail committee continued with the planned route. No one saw that coming.

A neighborhood in Post Falls, the Pinevilla subdivision, also opposed the trail route citing a potential rise in crime, litter, and the trail being an endangerment to children. They too would lobby the Post Falls High Way District and the City of Post Falls to stop or relocate the trail route. The trail route would connect schools, parks and points of interest to neighborhoods and that idea was vociferously unacceptable.

The trail committee entertained the idea of including an equestrian path adjacent to the pedestrian and bicycle trail. This created a lot of enthusiasm amongst horse owners. However, as the plans progressed and it was apparent the trail would also be placed in the road right-of-way in order to get through some residential and commercial areas. Adding horses within the same designated trail with walkers, runners, and bicyclists right next to vehicle traffic, added an element that was potentially dangerous. The trail committee decided to abandon an equestrian trail, which stirred feelings of being misled by the horse owners.

Entering Coeur d'Alene was also a bit difficult for the trail planners. Several options were explored to bring the trail through the city, with Northwest Boulevard presenting as the logical route. Although gaining access, the trail width narrowed to about three feet along the one-mile section. It was hazardous to bicyclists and runners, and more hazardous to those without

THE TRAIL THAT ALMOST WASN'T

experience, mixing with vehicle traffic. The heavy amount of vehicle traffic on Northwest Boulevard ran parallel to the trail. Runners and bicyclists were separated by a painted line, the fog line.

A physical barrier is ideal in separating pedestrians and vehicle traffic. At that time there were no sidewalks or other means of movement for pedestrians on this boulevard. This somewhat unsafe condition lasted over 10 years. The City of Coeur d'Alene rebuilt Northwest Boulevard in 2001, and the trail was not part of the new plan. Around that same time the W-I Forest Products site was purchased for the Riverstone Development. The purchaser of the lumber mill site was planning a subdivision promoted for live, work and play. He offered to allow the trail to pass through the subdivision, moving it off of Northwest Boulevard and closer to the Spokane River. This was easier said than done. A railroad issue arose stalling this movement for nearly 2 years.

Reaching eastward beyond Coeur d'Alene, trail enthusiasts expressed interest in what would soon become an abandoned four lane section of Interstate 90. The Idaho Transportation Department (ITD) would be relocating I-90 about ¼ mile away from the lake shoreline. Trail planners saw an opportunity to secure the lake side lane for the last five miles of the trail system. That idea had cold lake water thrown on it at our first inquiry. The Idaho Transportation Department would be abandoning the old interstate, but they intended to transfer jurisdiction to the East Side Highway District. ITD did not want to encumber the land with a pedestrian/bicycle trail. The highway district expressed no interest in the trail idea. Nearly three years later in 1990, a tragedy on the I-90 relocation project became a key turning point.

There were many historic and scenic views to incorporate into the trail concept and route. However, getting access across the river to these places became what appeared to be an insurmountable problem. Trail planners lacked funds to purchase a needed railroad right of way in Post Falls, and there was push back from residents about the use of the Corbin Ditch. Local mills and the Post Falls Highway District were going to oppose the trail route. A Post Falls neighborhood was up in arms over fear of how the trail would degrade and devalue their neighborhood. It also seemed as though there would not be support to go east beyond Coeur d'Alene using an abandoned highway lane.

Odds against this trail ever happening slammed deeply into the thoughts of the trail supporters. However, they were not willing to fold up the trail idea due to the rising issues. The trail concept and its benefits were greater than the concerns being expressed. Projecting ahead 20, 30, 50 years, they strongly believed that this trail project was worth working through the issues that seemed to be popping up so unexpectedly.

Chapter 2
A Movement

A movement taking place all across the country would be directly related to the popularity of trails. The subtle, but steady movement in American lifestyle changed the course of railroads and access to trails in America forever.

Over 150 years ago, our nation's governing body recognized the need to expand west, and expand rapidly. The United States Government issued land grants west of the Mississippi River, which encouraged mass migration from pioneers desiring to start a new life in America's expansive frontier. Wagon trains rolled west moving thousands of our ancestors making a difficult, and often times deadly journey.

Railroads quickly became the fastest way to move people, livestock and goods. Responding to the need to improve this mode of transportation, the U.S. Government assisted by issuing land grants, easements, and financial grants to expedite rail connectivity from coast to coast and border to border. The railroads reached their peak of becoming the nation's number one transporter around the 1920's. Over 275,000 miles of railroad tracks crisscrossed the country as people and freight moved in mass. The railroads fueled the economy of a fast-growing nation and stood out as the premiere mode of all transportation.

After the turn of the twentieth century, production of the automobile gave the first indication that things would not remain the same for much longer. Americans thrived on independence, and a strong desire to move about their town, their state, and their country. By the 1920's automobiles were quite common, and affordable, thanks in part, to Henry Ford. The Model T could be bought for less than $400, and it gave people that increased sense of freedom. It was not a very comfortable, or reliable way to travel, but millions purchased the Model T.

Henry Ford was once quoted as saying, "The Model T may never be replaced, it is all we need, and I will paint your Model T in any color of your choice as long as it is black." However, even that would not remain the same for long. In 1928, the Model T gave way to the Model A, and change again occurred rapidly. The new automobile drove forward as the favorite way to move about the land. Roads, in that day, were unpaved, potholed, and often muddy. Going great distances was a challenge, but that too would improve before the middle of the century.

At this time, the railroads began to lose their two-handed grip on the transportation market. As the automobile revolution rapidly improved, the trucking industry also experienced sweeping changes. Larger trucks with more payload began to haul supplies that were once moved exclusively by railroad. Trucks could deliver products directly to manufacturers and distributors quickly, and in large quantity.

The auto and truck industries paralleled the rise of another new industry, aviation. By the middle of the century, air travel stepped ahead of the railroads as the quickest way for people to move throughout the country. The airplane industry expanded to move both people and cargo faster than the railroads, cars or trucks.

By the end of World War II, a national hero had risen, General Dwight D. Eisenhower, Commander of the Allied Forces on the European Front. After the war in 1950, he was elected to the presidency. He put in motion another revolution. President Eisenhower wanted Interstate Highways connecting all the major cities throughout the country. It was rumored, he formed this plan to create a great highway system which would allow for massive troop deployment anywhere in the country, should America ever be invaded.

Eisenhower's planned Interstate highway system was also rumored to be able to accommodate transport planes that could use those highways, if need be. The even numbered interstates would run east and west with the numbering system starting in the south and increasing northward. Odd numbered interstates would run north and south with the lowest number beginning in the west and higher numbers towards the east. President Eisenhower's goal was to connect America through an Interstate highway system that would keep America moving and boost its economy. He often commented on the European highway systems that he saw during WWII, which were designed to move vehicles quickly with little to no restrictions, including no speed limits in some places.

The movement that was about to sweep across the nation was all but in place. Automobiles, long haul trucks, and airplanes had taken a huge part of the transportation market away from the railroads. The change was so dramatic that from the 1960's and into the 1980's the railroads abandoned tracks by the thousands of miles. Those deserted railroad lines however, were still being used with a slightly different purpose. People were walking the abandoned railroad lines to explore, discover, and marvel at the bridges and tunnels that the railroads had so expertly constructed.

The U.S. Congress became concerned about the high number of rail corridors being vacated, and in 1983 introduced a bill for 'Rail Banking'. The National Trail Systems Act was designed to preserve old railroad corridors for future rail use by converting them to interim trails. Three years later the Rails to Trails Conservancy was formed, and trails have since become common (and necessary) in rural, urban and metropolitan areas. The movement that forever changed the use of abandoned railroad corridors had expanded to see a rise in demand for trail connectivity in towns and cities across America. The demand was not exclusive to railroad corridors, but would include roads and highways, and other integral connections making it safer and easier, for pedestrian and bicyclists to move around. [1]

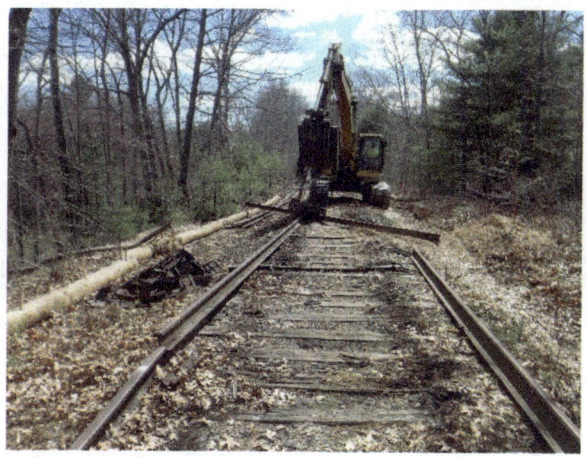

Rails to Trails Archive Photo

The North Idaho Centennial Trail embodied the cutting edge of this movement beginning in 1987, when the Centennial Trail concept was introduced to our area. It took nearly nine years to complete the trail as this movement had not been embraced by everyone in the community. A pedestrian trail connecting communities, cities, and two states was still a relatively new idea.

---

[1] www.american-rails.com 2016

Such change can be difficult to both introduce and to accept, not to mention pull off.

Chapter 3
Benefits of the Trail

The North Idaho Centennial Trail, a scenic, historic trail has far reaching, positive, benefits for the community. The big picture of the trail benefits includes impacts to vast areas such as economics, social interaction, recreation, transportation, and environmental preservation.

Many books and articles have been written on the economic impact of trails, parks and open space. It is often misunderstood or underrated; a problem that can be found from community to community. This failure to recognize, or unawareness of the benefits can extend to elected officials, their staff, as well as the general citizenry throughout the United States. That awareness is changing even though it seems to be slow.

Trails have been around for as long as people have been on the Earth. In the last 40 to 50 years the value a trail system brings to a community has stepped to the forefront in America. The value of open space and parks in England reaches back nearly 200 years. It was referenced as the 'Proximate Principle,' and addressed the phenomenon of property values being greater in proximity to public spaces.

This principle made its way to America in the early 1800's, but was overshadowed with the industrial revolution. Working hours were long and people were migrating to cities by the millions where the factories were being built. Housing was a problem as well as water supplies and sanitation.

The effects of the industrial revolution led to many labor laws being introduced and implemented. A few of the issues that arose were number of weekly working hours, collective bargaining, working conditions and perhaps most importantly, child labor laws. The industrial revolution spanned a time of nearly 100 years. Some historians say the industrial revolution began in America as early as the 1790's. Although it catapulted America into becoming an industrial powerhouse, pain, suffering and growth occurred along the way. Pedestrian trails and public outdoor recreation came up short as a priority during most of that time. [2]

The first park in the United States that was deliberately planned was Central Park in New York. Central Park was nothing more than swampland with trash, pigsties, squatters and slaughter houses. Reportedly, a pervasive and obnoxious odor emanated from the site. New York acquired the land in the 1850's and consulted with Frederick Olmsted on what the land could become.

Olmsted is considered the father of American landscape architecture. In the *Proximate Principle,* a book written by John L. Crompton (second addition, 2004), he points out that Olmstead employed the proximate principle to demonstrate how New York could buy the land without increasing taxes. New York dignitaries would debate with Olmstead that the highest and best use of the land was to convert it to high-end real estate. The city maintained that the Central Park land could add 10,000 homes to the tax base. [3]

Olmsted successfully demonstrated the relationship between public parks and real estate values. Central Park would be accessible to all New Yorkers and visitors, while the areas adjacent to the park become more

---

[2] Brooks, J. Rebecca. 2108 The Industrial Revolution in America
[3] Crompton L. John. 2004 The Proximate Principle

valuable due to the proximity to the grand park plan. The area immediately around the park became home to families like the Vanderbilt's and Rockefellers. Hotels and restaurants sprung up throughout the area. Central Park became an example of how parks enhance community values. John Crompton quotes the New York Parks Commission 25 years after the development of the park. *"The three wards adjacent to the park paid one dollar in every thirteen dollars the city received in taxes, but after the parks development they paid one-third of the entire expense of the city, even though acquiring the land for Central Park removed 10,000 lots from the city's tax roll."*

Converting open space into subdivisions is not the answer to improving a community's financial solvency. Long term planning with regard to the quality of life and health of a community should always be the highest priority. Many years later, the principle applied to open space and real estate would come front and center for trails and greenways.

Trail development gained interest across the country in the 1970's. A common concern that arose as trails began to pop up across the country is that residents believed a trail would attract criminal elements. This concern was coupled with decreasing property values and trash. One trail recently built was the Burke-Gilman Trail in Seattle, Washington. The Burke-Gilman trail is 12 miles long and was completed in 1979. It passes through neighborhoods, commercial areas and the University of Washington.

Studies on trails relating to the impact a trail was having on real estate values and crime had yet to be done. In 1987, Seattle evaluated the impact of the Burke-Gilman Trail. Eight years had passed since the trail was built, and it was thought that stakeholders would have formed a clear opinion on the trails effect on property. The authors of the report concluded: *"In summary, this study indicates that concerns about decreased property values, increased crime, and a lower quality of life due to the construction of multi-use trails is unfounded. The study indicates that multi-use trails are an amenity that helps sell homes, increases property values and improves the quality of life."* [4]

In the late 1990's the National Recreation and Parks Association contracted with Texas A & M University to research and report on the dynamics of the Proximate Principle. The result sparked a renewed interest in the Proximate Principle all across the nation. Specifically, the report identifies the increased property values derived from parks, open space, and trails, due to the close proximity to these assets. Higher property values and increased tax base result from this proximity.

It is estimated that trails in urban settings enhance property values of homes along, or near a trail, to be upwards of 4% to 12% higher than homes located farther away from trails. This is known as the 'Proximate Principle'. The closer the proximity, the higher the value. This is also true for homes near parks, water, and golf courses. People want to be located near a safe walking/bicycling route for leisure exercise, and for alternative commuting if the trail system provides connectivity to other destinations, such as a work place, or school. The North Idaho Centennial Trail does that.

Realtors, real estate agents, and real estate brokers are quick to recognize this benefit, and often point out the proximity of the trail in their advertising of a home for sale. A former member of the North Idaho Centennial Trail Foundation, and owner of Fortus

---

[4] www.burkegilmantrail Friends of the Burke Gilman Trail

Realty, Denise Lundy, compiled a list of sub-divisions that are next to, or close to, pedestrian and bicycle trails. There are approximately 35 sub-divisions in the community that benefit from their proximity to trail systems. Developers are getting better at recognizing this phenomenon, however some of them still need a meeting with someone, such as the author of this book, to fully understand and appreciate the long-term benefits.

In order to fully appreciate the value of this principle, an in-depth review of property values and comparisons by a professional business that operates in this field should be conducted. Another way to look at the benefits supporting a healthy tax base as a result of the proximate principle is to imagine if the assets were removed from the equation. What would the value of homes be if parks, open space, golf courses, and trails with esthetic views were removed? The tax base would be reduced significantly, and services that we take for granted such as police, fire, street service, and parks and recreation, to name a few, would be diminished. Our quality of life would change if these amenities did not exist.

This author would argue that the funds generated to the tax base as a direct result of these public amenities are not returned proportionately for the support, acquisition and development of these public outdoor amenities. Some would make the argument that the financial status of the governing agency would dictate that they cannot afford to allocate funds for these public amenities. I maintain they cannot afford not to.

The economic impact does not stop with homes, property values, and a healthy tax base. In a recent economic impact study funded by the North Idaho Centennial Trail Foundation, it revealed that nearly three million dollars ($3,000,000) in new money is brought into the community every year. This is a direct result of the North Idaho Centennial Trail, and events that are hosted on the trail. It is also important to note that some economists say that new money turns over in a community approximately 7 times before it leaves the community. [5]

The new money generated as a result of the Centennial Trail is distributed in a variety of places. Local businesses, such as hotels, restaurants, gas stations, souvenir shops, breweries, and coffee stands are just a few of the beneficiaries of trail events. These newly generated dollars help to pay wages, rents, mortgages, insurances, taxes, and hopefully, fun times, allowing the new dollars to be spent again and again.

The aforementioned $3,000,000 in new money brought into the community is generated from three events sponsored by the North Idaho Centennial Trail Foundation. These events, the Coeur d'Alene Marathon, Ales for the Trail, and Coeur d'Fondo are growing in popularity. They will lead to additional funds coming into the community on an annual basis. The City of Coeur d'Alene and the City of Post Falls also host events directly related to trail activities. Those events are estimated to generate additional new money, upwards of $6,000,000. Financially, the trail system has become a major part of the county's economic engine.

The social benefit of the Centennial Trail is also a major part of the community's overall health. The length of the Centennial Trail, 23-miles long, promotes community involvement, serves as a meeting place, and provides opportunities to interact with others.

---

[5] Peterson, Steven. Research Economist
2019 Economic Impact of the North Idaho Centennial Trail

Relationships are built, renewed, and enjoyed throughout the year. Residents along the trail use it frequently for exercise, walking the dog, walking and running with family and friends, pushing a stroller, using a wheelchair, taking a stroll, a bike ride, or to simply engage with the trail's availability and the environment. More importantly, trails and greenbelts are accessible to everyone and every age group.

Health and recreational benefits of a trail are immeasurable. A short stroll can lift your mood, get creative juices flowing, and perhaps, solve a problem. A recent study published in *Psychology Today* found that walking improved both convergent and divergent thinking, the two types associated with enhanced creativity.[6] We were not built to be sedentary, but to move, walk, or run. Activity increases your metabolism, and wards off the evils of high blood pressure, even diabetes. Walking on a trail does not require the cost of a membership. It does not even require specific clothing, and shoes can be optional. An individual can literally save money by walking on a trail, and reducing health care costs with a little bit of exercise every day, or a few times a week, thus creating a personal, and positive, health benefit and economic impact. Moving, walking, or running clears cortisol, the "stress hormone," out of your system, and also helps stop the never-ending stream of worries going through your mind, according to a study published in *The American Journal of Cardiology.*[7]

Trails have been introduced for many decades as an alternative mode of transportation. They serve as an important, if not crucial, element in an urban setting.

---

[6] Ward, Thomas Phd 2017 Psychology Today
[7] Galic, Bohana 2019 www.livstrong.com

THE TRAIL THAT ALMOST WASN'T

Many people will ride a bike to and from their work place, seeking to avoid congested streets and highways. With little vehicle interaction, The North Idaho Centennial Trail provides a safe alternative transportation corridor.

The linear design of a park and greenbelt serves to preserve the things that we enjoy, and too often take for granted. They help to preserve natural landscape areas that can include waterfront access points and/or viewpoints. Trails have a minimal environmental impact and a high degree of conservation.

In summary, the North Idaho Centennial Trail:
- increases the value of nearby properties.
- boosts spending at local businesses.
- makes the community a more attractive place to live, and vacation.
- influences business location and relocation decisions.
- reduces medical costs by encouraging exercise.
- provides alternative transportation.
- increases tax revenue.

The National Parks and Recreation Association uses this slogan about open spaces: ***The Benefits are Endless.*** That statement most accurately reflects the benefits of the North Idaho Centennial Trail.

Chapter 4
The Bridge

Crossing the Spokane River at state line, the railroad bridge was originally built by Milwaukee Railroad in 1910. Railroad companies that built bridges, trestles and tunnels took pride in the structural and engineering feats of these structures. This particular bridge work was better known for its pilings that are made of concrete and have an elongated oval shape. Three massive pilings support the steel girders of which the trains run across. The pilings at this location were built large enough to accommodate a second set of tracks, if ever necessary. A second set of tracks was never added at this crossing.

The last train to cross the bridge was in 1974. When trains were no longer scheduled to use this track, it was shut down, and the crossing was abandoned. The bridge was rendered inaccessible by the placement of dirt and barricades. It remained unused for more than a decade before the trail design team identified it as a viable pedestrian/bicycle access to cross the Spokane River between Idaho and Washington.

Once numerous, railroad companies in the 1980's were bought, or merged, with larger railroads. BNSF purchased land from other railroads and this particular bridge was part of larger acquisitions that spanned several states. Most of the railroad lines acquired by BNSF were still active. The inactive lines would be liquidated, or sold, like this bridge. [8]

Railroad companies hold vast amounts of land across the entire country; in many locations, the trains no

---

[8] www.burlingtonnorthernrailroad.com 2016

longer run through those areas. Their unused or abandoned rail lines are often put into the hands of land management companies, who sell the properties. This particular bridge, along with the property on both sides, was placed with Glacier Park, a land management company that liquidates railroad properties for BNSF. The railroads are required to submit a recommendation to the federal government before they can abandon their lines. That process can take a couple of years before the railroads are cleared to liquidate the land.

The crossing of the Spokane River at the border of two states became a substantial challenge. The Spokane trail organizers brought their trail to the state line. The river was in Idaho, so establishing a way to cross the river fell to Idaho. Burlington Northern Railroad and their land management company, Glacier Park, informed the trail organizers that they had a pending sale on the historic railroad bridge. This information led the trail organizers to diligently search for alternative routes.

Going north or south from the point where The Spokane River Centennial Trail would connect to the intersection of Spokane Bridge Road and Seltice Way was problematic. The roads were narrow with little to no right-of-way. If the trail was to travel east onto Seltice Way, it would encounter a vehicle bridge that was not built to accommodate pedestrians or bicycles. This route was unsafe and would take trail users further from the intended goal to be near the river. The trail organizers refocused on the abandoned railroad bridge even though that idea appeared to be a lost cause.

Numerous calls had already been placed to Glacier Park and to BNSF regarding the abandoned railroad bridge. Acme Concrete, the perspective buyer, was intending to use the bridge to move their equipment back and forth from Washington to Idaho in order to avoid using the Interstate. Construction was very brisk in the 1980's and it must have made sense for them to want to use this route.

It did not make sense to the trail enthusiasts. Construction had its high times and also had its low times. The current use of the bridge for construction transportation would fade, and the bridge would again sit unused. It would never sit unused if it was a pedestrian-bicycle trail. Bicycling started to emerge as an alternative mode of transportation, and there would be many more cyclists, runners and walkers that could use the bridge than construction equipment.

However, the reality and excitement of creating a legacy trail in North Idaho was starting to fade. Even though a lot of people had initially caught the vision of this project, pedestrian access across the Spokane River appeared to be an idea that would not reach fruition.

One last inquiry was to ask for advice from our congressional representative, Larry Craig. Sandy Patano served as the office manager and contact person for the congressman's Coeur d'Alene office. As parks director, I explained and summed up the dilemma; the trail project hovered in jeopardy due to the difficulty in crossing the Spokane River. Congressman Craig had expressed support for this phenomenal project earlier in the conceptual design stage. In 1988, he toured the proposed trail corridor with County Commissioner Evalyn Adams, and Post Falls Mayor Kent Helmer. The hope to acquire the abandoned railroad bridge, restore it, and use it as the bi-state crossing was shared with Sandy Patano. She was also made aware that it probably would not happen since BNSF appeared to have a pending sale on the bridge, thus potentially forcing the trail committee to abandon the project.

Ms. Patano shared that Congressman Craig was supportive of public outdoor recreation, including this trail project, and he was familiar with the history of the railroads. She promised to forward the information to the Congressman.

This visit buoyed the hopes of the trail organizers, albeit temporarily. Soon they wondered, *why would the Congressman concern himself with a pedestrian trail in Kootenai County?*

A few days passed since the discussion in Larry Craig's office, when an unexpected call came into the Coeur d'Alene Parks office. On the other end of the line was an executive from Glacier Park, Walter Ferrell. It seemed apparent by the tone of the conversation that the Centennial Trail Committee had become the proverbial thorn in his side. Mr. Ferrell simply asked, "What do you want?" The inflexion in the question was similar to that of a parent whose child had interrupted them 20 or 30 times. Yep, the trail folks had developed into a nuisance.

A million things raced through my mind while I was on the phone with Glacier Park, all the while displaying a wide smile. My foremost thought was that Representative Craig must have made a well-placed phone call to someone in the BNSF hierarchy, and this was the result. The opportunity to speak with Glacier Park and/or BNSF was what the trail planners needed.

The vision to develop a bi-state paved pedestrian trail that would allow the citizenry from two states to travel relatively un-impeded of vehicle conflicts was explained to Mr. Farrell. Acknowledging that BNSF and Glacier Park had a pending sale with Acme Concrete, the trail planners still wanted the opportunity to meet and talk with them personally about this bridge.

Walter Ferrell said he would mull this over and call back. The trail planners were pleasantly surprised when he did return the call. A meeting was scheduled for the following week in Spokane at the Burlington Northern/Glacier Park office.

A few days before the meeting, another unexpected call came into my CDA Parks office. This time it came from Mike Newell, a local real estate attorney. Mike said he had heard about the interest in acquiring the bridge for the purpose of building a trail and had been following that progress. He heard about the pending meeting in Spokane and asked if he could be of assistance. We absolutely welcomed and appreciated his help.

Mike Newell, Randy Haddock (trail committee co-chair), and myself attended the railroad bridge meeting in Spokane. There we met with five BNSF/Glacier Park executives convened in the conference room. Introductions took place without the exchange of much pleasantries.

The hopeful trail reps took the opportunity to explain the purpose for requesting the meeting. The vision of a bi-state trail was again described in detail. The emphasis was on the need to acquire the railroad bridge. Without the bridge, the bi-state project would most likely fizzle out. They listened and thanked the trail representatives for being there. Reiterating that because of their pending sale with Acme Concrete, they could not be of any help for the ambitious project.

There was a long silence as Mike, Randy and I pondered this latest, and certainly, final rejection. The vision of this trail project had momentarily materialized, and then again, all but disappeared.

However, Attorney Mike Newell studied the folks from BNSF and Glacier Park sitting across the table and asked if they had reviewed the Idaho Statutes on liquidating property over water controlled by the state. After a long moment of silence, Mike explained that the statute of one state can be quite different from that of another state on this issue. The construction of the bridge began only after a permit from the Idaho Department of Lands (IDOL) was issued. The IDOL owned the land under the water, and everything that happened over the water can only be approved by the State of Idaho. The bridge over the water, as well as the land below the water, was controlled by that state. The proposed sale to Acme Concrete would change the intended use of the bridge, and that would trigger the need for a renewed easement permit from the State of Idaho addressing these reversionary issues.

An easement was granted to the railroad in 1910, but it was not a permanent easement. If and when changes of use occur, a new easement application would be required. Mike added that perhaps the first right of refusal should be offered to the local municipality in Idaho, or Kootenai County. He continued to explain that while Washington State may differ, the bridge and the adjoining property on both sides of the bridge are in Idaho.

The meeting ended at that point. The trail representatives were told that BNSF and Glacier Park would consider the points raised in the discussion.

The following week, I received a call from Mr. Ferrell at the Glacier Park office. The message was that the pending sale of the bridge had been withdrawn. The sale of the bridge, and adjoining acreage on both sides could be purchased for the Centennial Trail at the same price; $180,000. This was truly a highpoint in the trail development process. It seemed incredible to think this worthwhile project was nearly shut down, but now was newly revived by the opportunity to acquire the essential railroad bridge.

As parks director, I had once compared the acquisition of the bridge to that of a championship baseball game. "Top of the ninth, two outs, runner on first, and we are down by one run in a loser goes home game. Emerging from the dugout comes a pinch-hitter; Congressman Craig. He steps up to the plate, digs in his cleats, and on the first pitch – WHAM! He hits one out of the park. A U. S. Congressman stepped up, made a phone call on behalf of the trail project, which put us back in the game. But it wasn't over yet. The deal still needed to be closed. Relief pitcher, Mike Newell was called upon next. Mike walked onto the field and very adeptly put the sale of the bridge into perspective with respect to Idaho, causing the former deal to be reconsidered in favor of the trail. The Centennial Trail will move on to the next chapter of this exciting trail project".

After all the elation, there was a major reality check; the $180,000 was not in the coffers to buy the bridge. Land acquisition had not been factored into the budget. But that could not be a deterrent. I thought about the acquisition process including land appraisals, public hearings, and identifying funding. However, I decided that should not be a discussion to have with Glacier Park, and the acquisition of this bridge should move forward with every expectation that it will happen. Without any financial authority to do so I, as the Coeur d'Alene Parks Director, accepted the offer to buy the bridge. Walter Ferrell said he would have the papers drawn up for the sale.

The City of Coeur d'Alene, the City of Post Falls, and Kootenai County, the respective powers-to-be in this project, could not afford to buy the bridge. Even the three of them together could not afford to share the cost. Surprisingly, when the three entities were informed of the pending bridge purchase that they might be committed to, there was very little, if any, concern about the bridge acquisition. Everyone involved recognized that the success of this trail project hinged on getting this bridge. Still, there was no money to seal the deal.

Governor Andrus was contacted about the need for $180,000. Although he was appreciative of the efforts and supported the trail project, the state did not have 180K either.

Walter Farrell from Glacier Park called the CDA parks office a few weeks later, saying they were preparing the documents for the sale and transfer of the bridge and the land. He requested a copy of the Idaho State Statute referencing the first right of refusal should be offered to the local municipality.

I told Mr. Farrell I would send him a copy. Next, I asked the City Attorney, if he would look up the statute and send over a copy. Later that afternoon, the city attorney called back to report he could not find the statute, but one of his assistants was going to the Gonzaga Law Library the next day, and he would get a copy.

The next afternoon, the City Attorney called again and said his assistant could not locate the statute in the law library. He suggested contacting Mike Newell to get the statute number so they could readily access it.

Upon contacting Mike and letting him know what was needed, he responded with a short expletive. Mike explained that a lot of information was imparted on the railroad execs, and unfortunately, they focused on the one topic that is not a law. There was no first right of refusal statute pertaining to the liquidation of railroad property in Idaho. However, the railroad, and/or buyer of the bridge, would have to go through the permitting process with the State of Idaho to buy or sell the property. He added the process might be a challenge for them.

The challenge for BNSF and Acme Concrete would come from pressure the trail organizers would put upon BNSF and Acme Concrete by requesting the state (IDOL) deny a new or revised use permit for the bridge. The trail organizers believed their plan to be a better use of the abandoned railroad bridge. They would ask IDOL to consider the long historic transportation use of the bridge, and to have it remain in public transportation use, such as the proposed pedestrian and bicycle trail. Hundreds of thousands of people could use this corridor versus very few construction vehicles by comparison.

The response back to the railroad regarding their request for the state statute was not done in a timely fashion. In fact, a response to the request never happened. Fortunately, a U. S. Congressman intervened on behalf of the trail project, opening up a needed dialogue with the railroads.

Attorney Mike Newell, further engaged BNSF's attention by identifying potential reversionary issues that would assuredly be raised by the Department of Lands and the State of Idaho. The U. S. Congress had passed bills establishing the Rails to Trails Initiative that had occurred only a few short years earlier in 1983 and 1986. There were other recent congressional acts that BNSF may have considered in their decision to withdraw from the sale of this bridge to a private party and offer to sell it for trail use.

Believing the bridge would be secured, the process of developing design documents began in earnest. The focus started with the construction of the trail's first 5

THE TRAIL THAT ALMOST WASN'T

miles, from the state line to Spokane Street in Post Falls. This included restoring the railroad bridge.

Work on the bridge started in late 1989, less than a year after the acquisition discussions. The bridge reconstruction was completed one year later in 1990. The first five miles of the trail was opened and celebrated in October of that year. An issue that did not get resolved regarding the bridge acquisition popped up a few years later as quite a surprise.

In 1993, three years after the first section of Trail was officially dedicated and opened, a message came from Glacier Park thanking the Idaho trail planners for making 'their' bridge look good. The Spokesman Review ran a story on the issue with the headlines saying that the "Centennial Trail Bridge borders on illegal." What did that even mean, the bridge borders on *illegal*?

Quite a few issues along the 23-mile trail corridor persisted, some quite contentious. Those issues distracted the trail organizers, and the county, from following up on the sale closure of the railroad bridge crossing. It was wrongly assumed by the trail organizers that the county was following up on this transaction, likewise the county assumed the trail organizers were doing the follow up. The transaction to transfer ownership did not happen and BNSF still owned the bridge.

DAMAGE CONTROL. The Trail Committee had not yet identified where the $180,000 could come from to buy the bridge and adjoining land. Neither the county nor the trail committee had received a statement for the bridge purchase from Glacier Park.

Letters were sent back and forth between the county, the trail committee, and Glacier Park, assuring the sale and purchase from both parties. Bob Nelson, co-chair of the Kootenai County Centennial Committee and the first chair of the newly formed North Idaho Centennial Trail Foundation, took on the arduous task of closing the transaction.

Surprise, the property deed finally arrived in 1993, nearly five years after the initial discussions. Further surprise, the deed came as a gift. The land and bridge were being transferred to the North Idaho Centennial Trail Foundation for the sum of ten dollars ($10.00). It is unknown if perhaps Congressman Craig requested that the bridge be donated to the foundation, due to all the United States Government had done to help the railroads over the past 150 years. Or, if the railroad recognized the best use for the bridge was exactly what the trail committee had intended, and/or what they had done with it. The railroad bridge was restored and railroad history would live on. It is not known why they gifted the bridge to the foundation but everyone involved was certainly appreciative and celebrated the gift.

Shortly after the bridge was deeded to the North Idaho Centennial Trail Foundation in 1993, the foundation officially recorded it at the Kootenai County Courthouse. Within a few months of the land being recorded in the name of the North Idaho Centennial Trail Foundation, the Board of County Commissioners notified the Trail Foundation that they could not legally own property and needed to transfer the ownership of the bridge to the county. The transfer of bridge ownership from the NICTF to Kootenai County then occurred.

The NICTF Board had not verified the issue of land ownership. The notification from the county that the foundation could not own property was inaccurate. A 501 (c) 3 foundation, such as the NICTF, can own property and there are greater benefits to have them own, and hold land for public use. The foundation can generate sponsorship fees related to the historical bridge. The county, on the other hand, possessed restrictions on sponsorships and commercial advertising.

An unexpected event, and a fun one, began with a call to the trail committee from the Washington and Idaho Surveyors Association in 1989. They wanted to participate in this trail development project by re-surveying the state line, and doing it with equipment and attire from that earlier era. The line separating the two states was drawn in 1873 by Surveyor Rollie J. Reeves. The association members utilized an 1870's Solar Transit to retrace Rollie's steps along two miles of the state line. They found the 1873 surveying to be quite accurate. A 40,000-ton boulder was placed on the state line with a plaque commemorating those efforts and dedicating the Centennial Trail. The boulder was situated on the west side of the historic railroad bridge.

Another brief note on this bridge; In 1990, the Idaho Department of Lands was contacted by Kootenai County to renew the bridge permit over the water. The trail design included plans to completely refurbish the bridge and convert its use from railroad transportation to a pedestrian and bicycle trail. The State of Idaho permitted the planned, new use in October of 1990. Mike Newell was quite right with his prediction of the permitting process. Burlington Northern Railroad, and Acme Concrete would have had a more difficult time securing a new permit.

The stars that had all but flickered out started to shine brightly on this part of the trail. Unfortunately, new situations began to crop up, causing things to grow worse as the trail project headed eastward from the Idaho/Washington state line.

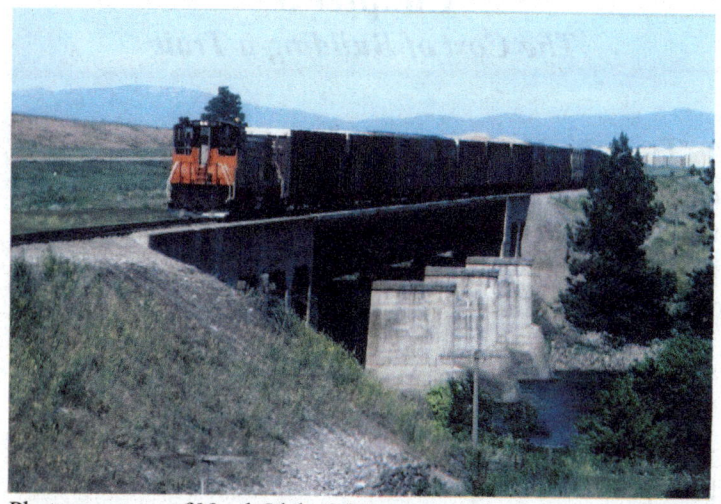

Photo courtesy of North Idaho Museum

This may have been the last trains to cross the railroad bridge, and the Spoken River, at the state line. Burlington Northern Santa Fe Railroad closed the bridge in 1974.

Chapter 5
The Cost of Building a Trail

The North Idaho Centennial Trail was estimated to cost $2.4 Million Dollars in 1987. This cost was one of the highest for outdoor public recreation endeavors that had been proposed in the community to date. This cost would nearly double after an unexpected incident in 1990. The cost was higher for the 39 miles of trail in Washington; they were needing $5.9 Million Dollars. The combined trail projects for Idaho and Washington, were estimated to be $8.3 million dollars in 1987. This trail project would become the focus of an incredible event.

The vision of this trail grew rapidly, getting support, and attention from our state's respective federal legislators. They were approached by people from both states asking if there was an opportunity for us to seek federal funding. Tom Foley, the Speaker of the House, held a position which wielded a lot of authority and responsibility. He was an elected representative from Washington and member of The Democrat Party. Another House member, Larry Craig, a Republican, was sent to Washington, D.C. by the people of Idaho.

Representatives Foley and Craig took time to visit their states' respective trail routes and ask questions. The congressmen were being asked to request federal funds on behalf of Washington and Idaho to assist with the trail development. Both men recognized that a debate would likely occur on the house floor as a result of this funding request.

Representative Craig introduced the budget request for partial funding of the bi-state trail project. Speaker Foley endorsed the request. It was approved by the

House of Representatives and forwarded to the U.S. Senate as part of the 1988-89 Fiscal Budget.

The budget process takes quite a while to get through the House and Senate, and then onto the President for his signature. This year was no different, and even though this bi-state request was miniscule in the overall federal budget, it was huge to the trail planners from both states. We followed the federal budget process like it was the Super Bowl.

Soon, another trail ally stepped into the picture, Jim McClure, United States Senator and chairman of the Senate Appropriations Committee. Senator McClure was sent to Washington D.C. by Idaho citizens and was also a member of the Republican Party. When the budget leaves the House and goes to the Senate it gets another thorough review by various Senate committees. Our request rested with Senator McClure's Appropriations Committee. Fortunately, this project was recognized by Representatives and Senators from both states as having a long-term importance to their respective communities, serving social, health and economic purposes.

With Senator McClure's help, the request survived the Senate and was included in the 1988-89 Federal budget when President Ronald Regan approved and signed it. This appropriation did not fund the project in its entirety, contributing only a bit more than 50% of the needed amount. Idaho received $1.35M of the needed $2.4M, and Washington received $3.1M of their needed $5.9M. The purpose of restricting the request to approximately 50%, required the local communities to commit to raising the rest of the funds; thereby demonstrating ownership of the project. The federal appropriation did not allow for land acquisition, personnel, or equipment. The funds were to be used for trail construction exclusively.

This financial accomplishment was incredible, nearly miraculous. First of all, it moved the project within reach of financial goals. Secondly, this was accomplished with the greatest amount of cooperation from both political parties. Usually on opposite sides of an issue, they recognized the real value and worked together as one unit, a truly non-partisan project.

The federal allocation placed the project half-way to the goal, a huge boost to commitment and fund-raising efforts resulted. Trail enthusiasts in both states were ecstatic, and up for the challenge of raising the remaining funds.

As trail committee chairman, I believed the project would easily come to fruition now that the majority of funding had been allocated. I felt this to be a good time to step aside from the trail project, let others see it to completion, so I could spend more time on the duties of my other jobs at the CDA Parks Department. The trail project required daily involvement up to this point and the trail committee had people who could bring this project to closure. It had been beneficial to have a staff person in front of this project as a contact and spokesperson for the project. However, I announced to the trail committee at the end of June, 1988 that I would be stepping aside.

That did not go over as well as I expected. Recognizing that the project had become time consuming, Randy Haddock said he would work as co-chairperson with me.

Lance Bridges from Post Falls, brought forth the most convincing argument for me not to step aside. Lance was experiencing frequent calls and/or visits from a Pinevilla resident claiming that the trail was an irresponsible idea and should not be placed near a neighborhood or a school. He said he would like to put in more time on the project, but is dealing with enough issues in Post Falls. Lance believed we were a good team and to lose the lead contact at this point would create a burden for someone else. Those conversations led to a retracting of the decision to step aside. Hours spent on the trail project would get longer, and the project would become increasingly more difficult. But, for the time being, the team stayed intact and moved forward.

Several fund-raising ideas were discussed and implemented. Fund raising for any project encounters high and low points, and this one was no different. The trail committee experienced some rejections to secure funds. One of those was with the U. S. Forest Service. They awarded grants for pilot bridge projects of which the trail committee sought a $30,000 grant. They did not get it. The county, on behalf of the trail, requested that the Idaho Transportation Department, ITD, compensate the county for placing 650,000 cubic yards of fill material into the lake near Higgins Point for an Interstate on-ramp. That request was rejected. The state, at the encouragement of the governor, was petitioned for a portion of the Stripper Well Funds that Idaho had recently received from the Federal Government. Those funds did not materialize either. The trail committee did, however, sell hundreds of t-shirts, and sweatshirts that had the Centennial Trail logo silk-screened on them. The Coeur d'Alene Press became a corporate sponsor and did all of the advertising for the fund-raising efforts, other trail contributors included:
- Washington Water Power (now Avista) donated $5,000.
- The trail committee held a Hole-in-One Golf Tournament.

THE TRAIL THAT ALMOST WASN'T

- The Adjutant Company, run by Gordon Crow, was hired to expand the fund-raising activities, and they introduced the Centennial Trail monument that is located at the Independence Point Park area. The cost of having a name on the monument was $150 per line.
- Tidyman's Grocery, and Pepsi Cola teamed up, and donated a percentage of all Pepsi sales to the trail in the summer of 1988.
- A grant from the Department of Water Resources was awarded to acquire the $139,000, nearly 3-mile, Burlington Northern Railroad right of way in Post Falls.
- Coeur d'Alene High School Students initiated a 'Mile of Quarters' campaign. Quarters laid down side by side for one mile generated nearly $16,000.00.
- Panhandle Kiwanis had custom made benches installed along the designated trail route through the CDA City Park.
- Trail committee members sold t-shirts and sweat shirts raising nearly $10,000.

By 1989 the trail committee had raised, or had commitments, in excess of $250,000. Fund raising was looking good and the project, from the supporter's view, appeared more and more like it would become a reality. Businesses and individuals received trail recognition sponsorship plaques for significant donations.

At that time, a growing and somewhat quiet resistance to the trail route and trail concept became apparent. The task of securing funding and routing appeared to be so overwhelming that those in opposition to the trail likely felt there was nothing to be concerned about because this project was doomed from the beginning. Adversaries to the project could no longer wait and hope that the project would just go away. The intensity of the opposition surfaced and impacted local politics, rallied businesses (mostly lumber mills), and residents. It managed to halt expenditure of the federal appropriation, forcing the trail construction to stop. Months and months of debate and allegations ensued from the trail opposition efforts.

Chapter 6
Corbin Ditch

The Corbin Irrigation Ditch was created to bring water into the Spokane Valley from the head gate on the Spokane River in the City of Post Falls. The purpose was to make the land more fertile for farming as well as more valuable. Daniel C. Corbin financed the development of the irrigation ditch, or canal as it was called. Mr. Corbin was a railroad and mining magnate at that time.

The engineering of the ditch was done by W.L. Benham, who was connected to the Great Northern Railway. Work began on the ditch in 1899 and continued for nearly a decade. The irrigation ditch ran for nearly 30 miles into the Spokane Valley. It had several lateral ditches that totaled more than 50 miles, providing water to thousands of acres of mostly apple orchards. The Corbin Irrigation Canal was nearly 10 feet deep with a flat bottom almost 8 feet wide. The sides of the canal angled away from the bottom making the upper width of the canal nearly 15 feet wide. The mere size of the canal indicates it could move a lot of water for agriculture irrigation purposes. The ditch was abandoned in the 1940's as repairs became too costly and newer methods of delivering water were more effective. [9]

This historic ditch is still visible today in the Post Falls area adjacent to the Centennial Trail just west of Spokane Street. The last remnant of this historic canal is close to the area where it originated in 1899. Only a short section of the Corbin Ditch remains as most of the

---

[9] Houda, Kegan 2005. The Corbin Ditch – Spokane Historical

historic canal has been filled in by adjoining property owners west of this visible location.

Daniel Corbin left his footprint in other parts of the area as well. He brought in the Spokane to Coeur d'Alene electric railroad. Daniel Corbin owned several railroads and had his hands in farming and mining throughout Washington and Idaho. Some historians credited Danial Corbin for the growth and success of the Spokane area, largely due to his desire to make Spokane a railroad hub for transporting crops, ores and people. He is also credited with building a house on the southwest tip of Tubbs Hill in Coeur d'Alene. The foundations to that house are still visible today.

The Corbin Canal, or 'Ditch', was proposed to become part of the Centennial Trail experience by converting several miles of the ditch into a pedestrian trail. The ditch was not wide enough to accommodate pedestrians and bicycles. The two-wheel enthusiasts would use another paved trail immediately north of the Corbin Ditch. The trail committee was negotiating with Burlington Northern Railroad for the purchase of the abandoned railroad corridor that ran immediately north of the canal.

At one of the first informational meetings, the trail supporters were a bit surprised by the response of the residents near the Corbin Ditch with regard to their fears of what trail users might do to their property. They expressed concerns that trail users would trespass, leaving litter, and dog waste, and potentially de-value their property. It was agreed upon at that meeting not to pursue the Corbin Ditch as part of the trail corridor.

The abandoned railroad property that ran on the north side of the Corbin Ditch became the focus for the trail. The railroad right of way had widths ranging from 60 feet to 100 feet. This abandoned rail corridor was wide enough to accommodate the trail for a variety of users. That appeased the residents and that meeting ended on a positive note. The railroad offered the abandoned 3-mile section of right-of-way adjacent to the Corbin Ditch for $139,000.00. The trail committee responded promptly with a notice of intent to purchase.

The City of Post Falls took the lead on raising funds for the purchase of this railroad right-of-way. The Land & Water Conservation Fund (LWCF) surfaced as the most likely source of funds for this acquisition. The LWCF is a federally funded grant that is financed through off-shore oil leases. The government began leasing sites along the continental shelf in the 1960's. The leases were profitable to the government, and congress determined that the funds should be returned for the acquisition and preservation of public lands.

Interest from the LWCF's is distributed to the individual states and U.S. owned territories. The amount of those funds are determined by population. The state of Washington, with eight million people would receive a larger percentage of the funds than Idaho with two million population. An example of how beneficial the LWCF is to the state of Idaho and local communities, approximately 40% of the CDA park system was financed by this fund. Post Falls, Rathdrum and Hayden have all benefited from the LWCF.

The LWCF's are allocated annually to each of the respective states and territories. Each of those entities oversee the distribution and use of the funds with oversight from the National Park Service. The Idaho Department of Parks and Recreation is the agency that manages the LWCF allocation for Idaho. State park departments are almost exclusively the overseers of this federal funding source. Interestingly, the state does not have to share the funds with cities and counties. The state can use the funds to further their needs of improving state parks or acquiring needed land. Idaho chose to share the funds. Grant requests are considered in odd years for cities and counties and even years for state and other federal agencies. Kudos to the Idaho Parks & Recreation Department for including all of Idaho in this funding opportunity.

Unfortunately, Post Falls did not make the final cut on the LWCF for the acquisition of the railroad right-of-way. Another funding source did materialize through the Idaho Department of Water Resources. Kootenai County was the recipient of the $139,000 grant. Letters between Kootenai County and the Department of Water Resources confirmed the grant award. There is no indication that this source ever materialized again for other local projects or land acquisitions in Kootenai County.

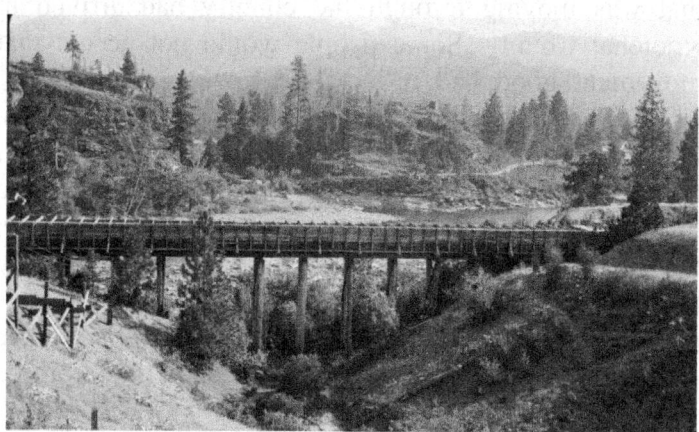

Photo courtesy of North Idaho Museum

The Corbin Canal brought water to the Rathdrum Prairie and the Spokane Valley for the purpose of expanding agriculture in this area. This photo shows the canal when it was fully operational around 1910.

Chapter 7
Trouble in the Hood

In early 1989, the first five miles of the trail from the State Line to Spokane Street in Post Falls gained approval for construction. However, the trail development would be faced with some very formidable opposition along other sections of the corridor. A growing concern was surfacing with regard to the perceived negative impact this trail project would have on the community. The mere suggestion of changing from the way things have always been, and adding something different, can cause a reaction with some people that do not want anything to change. The Centennial Trail project was encroaching into their space. The phenomenon of trails, and trail connectivity, that was moving through the country had arrived in Kootenai County. Some people would not accept that movement, good, bad, or indifferent.

Residents of a Post Falls neighborhood, Pinevilla, had circulated a petition to stop the trail from being built near their neighborhood. Those petitions were forwarded on to the Kootenai County Commissioners, the Post Falls City Council and the Post Falls Highway District. The trail route grew quite contentious in this part of Post Falls. Statements made portrayed the trail as one of the worst ideas and proposals perpetrated on the residents of the community.

The proposed and adopted route of the trail would run along Ponderosa Boulevard on the south side of this neighborhood from Ross Point Road to Greensferry Road. Part of the neighborhood was on the west side of Ross Point Road in Post Falls, and part of the neighborhood was on the east side of Ross Point Road just outside the Post Falls city limits in Kootenai County. These residents appealed to the City of Post Falls to stop the construction of the trail route. The geographic diversity of this neighborhood placed them in different electoral districts for Post Falls, and Kootenai County. However, all the residents were in the Post Falls Highway District, and that district became the primary lobbying arena.

Concerned residents from the neighborhood presented the Post Falls City Council, the Kootenai County Commissioners, and the Post Falls Highway District with a petition of over 300 signatures opposing the trail. When they presented this petition to the Post Falls City Council, they expressed that the trail would "open up the neighborhood to noise and trash unlimited." They went on to add that "they do not want these people in their neighborhood." A new and interesting debate was in full swing about having a pedestrian trail in Kootenai County.

A great deal of research had been conducted concerning public trail impact in other communities throughout Washington and Oregon. Property values and crime were major concerns for residents at the time trail concepts were being discussed in Oregon and Washington.

The Burke-Gillman Trail in Seattle was built in the late 1970's. Seattle conducted a survey regarding this trail in the mid 1980's. The study found that crime rates went down, property values went up, and people were choosing to live in close proximity to the trail.

Corvallis, Oregon was also well known for their network of trails, and how the community embraced and enjoyed the trail system. Other communities that had developed trails were contacted by the Centennial Trail committee for their findings on the pros and cons of a trail system. The results were mostly positive about trails being good for a community, citing such things as property values increasing and crime rates decreasing.

Closer to home, and one year earlier, The Spokesman Review reported that the Jacklin Seed Company was considering a request from the trail committee. The request concerned building the trail along the river immediately after crossing the historic railroad bridge. Jacklin Seed was developing the Riverbend Commerce Park, which fronted the Spokane River. Jacklin hired John Graham and Associates, a Seattle-based land planning group to help them with the development. These experts recommended that Jacklin Seed pursue the request from the trail committee. "Trails add to an industrial development and marketability," John Graham said. Duane Jacklin, President of Jacklin Seed, stated that they had been moderately opposing the Centennial Trail. Graham's report recommended that Jacklin seed change their perspective on trails. The report went on to say that "jogging and trails would be in the long-term interest for Riverbend."

The findings from Oregon, Washington, and the Jacklin report were also presented to the folks opposing the Centennial Trail. Still, they responded by saying *they don't care what happens in Seattle or elsewhere, they do not want a trail near them.* Efforts to stop the trail project, and routing, continued through the summer with escalating comments about the harm the trail would do if built within walking distance of neighborhoods.

At a public meeting on August 10, 1989, one Pinevilla resident told the County Commissioners, "The trail will run within two blocks of her house, but more importantly, it will run in front of the Ponderosa Elementary School. Running a major Interstate Urban Bike Trail past an elementary school is irresponsible and outrageous." The audience was hearing that the Centennial Trail would be harmful to children. Opposition grew along the trail route and more trail foes took up the cause to stop, or relocate, the Centennial Trail. The tactic to create a sense of this project as not being good for the community was getting some traction. Statements from anti-trail activists made to the media and elected officials, albeit inaccurate, were becoming increasingly difficult for people in the middle of the debate to separate facts from non-facts.

The trail committee found themselves dealing with assumptions that the trail would bring crime to a neighborhood, lower property values, attract the wrong kind of people to the community, and endanger children. Trail opponents also envisioned noise and trash everywhere. Coupling these unfounded fears with the highway district stating the proposed trail did not have right-of-way approval, and a trail design some considered ill-conceived from the beginning, should have been enough to make most people simply abandon the trail project.

Something was wrong and the trail committee members could not put their finger on the problem. Trail opponents were getting people to sign a petition by the hundreds against the trail, or trail location. Those who were promoting a petition probably believed that their concerns were real even though those concerns could not be supported by any data.

It is estimated that nearly half the population is uncomfortable with change. The Centennial Trail, albeit a new idea to this area, was creating a sense of uncertainty. Uncertainty can cause reason and logic to fly out the window. People can see change as an inherent risk. The risk of things not getting better, but worse. Those concerned, or afraid of change, personified the saying, "Better the devil you know than the devil you don't know." [10] We could supply all the data and results of other trails benefiting a community but that was not going to be enough for everyone to believe us. Both sides remained polarized on the issues.

The trail plan had, in fact, already taken all the issues and alternative routes into consideration. Numerous trail studies, already conducted in other areas, contradicted the issues/concerns raised by those opposing the Centennial Trail. Those against the trail refused to hear what trail studies said from other communities. Surprisingly, and frustratingly, the reasons the alternative routes would not work were not being considered by the opposition to the trail. The Highway District offered two other roads in their jurisdiction that they said they would approve; Poleline Avenue and /or Prairie Avenue. It was not difficult to address these alternatives and explain why they were both poor choices for the Centennial Trail.

The Post Falls City Council gave final approval to the routing through their community after several public hearings were held on that topic. In late summer of 1989, the city council had previously heard the concerns of the Pinevilla residents, who suggested alternative routing which would move the trail north and outside the city limits. The council reviewed and evaluated the pros and cons of the trail and trail routing. They were informed by the trail designer, Jon Mueller, that "relocating the trail away from residential areas would greatly decrease the use and accessibility of the trail, creating greater vehicle and pedestrian conflicts, as well as negating the purpose of installing the trail.

---

[10] Kanter, Rosabeth Moss 2012 Change Management

Relocating the trail would also affect costs, which the design team estimated to be an additional $800,000".

The Post Falls City Council voted to allow the trail to remain on the proposed route. Shortly after their decision to approve the trail route, vandalism occurred on the trail corridor at Ponderosa Boulevard in the Pinevilla Subdivision. Graffiti was spray painted on the street with non-sensical comments about the Centennial Trail.

The next very contentious area became Seltice Way. The opposition on that route included the Post Falls Highway District, Idaho Forest Industries, W-I Forest Products and Central Pre-Mix. There were four more lumber mills along the Spokane River, or within close proximity to the river or near Seltice Way. They too, joined the opposition to the trail location.

The Coeur d'Alene Press picked up on an interesting dichotomy of trail perception between residents of Post Falls, and Coeur d'Alene. In a Raspberries column on July 4, 1989, they noted that while some Post Falls residents were signing a petition by the hundreds to keep the trail out of their community, Coeur d'Alene residents were thrilled about having the historic trail pass by their homes. Some CDA residents were inquiring about installing benches and shrubbery to enhance the enjoyment of the trail.

By the spring of 1990, opposition to the trail routing past Pinevilla continued to be an issue. Post Falls Mayor, Kent Helmer, contacted Potlach Lumber, which was situated on the east side of Greensferry and stretched to Spencer Street. This section stretched half the distance between Greensferry and Ross Point Road. Using this section would allow for the trail to be routed on the south side of the Potlatch property, resolving the issue of taking the trail down Ponderosa Boulevard. The other half of the trail route, extending beyond the Potlatch property, would travel in a right of way controlled by the company of Idaho Veneer. This company produced large volumes of plywood products. Both businesses were serviced by Union Pacific Railroad. The railroad right-of-way width appeared to be wide enough to separate the trail from the lumber company service areas.

Mayor Helmer expressed in another Press article in April that his meetings with the Potlatch Lumber mill administration were positive, and they were receptive to the idea. However, this plan was ultimately rejected, and the original trail routing remained as the approved route.

Phase I of the trail came under construction from the state line to Spokane Street in Post falls, while a 'circling of the wagons' in opposition to the trail was in full swing along Seltice Way.

Chapter 8
The Fight Over Old Highway 10

Seltice Way, formerly Old Highway 10, became the ultimate battle ground for the Centennial Trail. The line in the sand had been drawn, and the trail supporters were told by the Post Falls Highway District that there was 'no way' they would be allowed to bring the trail down Seltice Way as they had planned.

Highway 10 was, at one time, the main highway between CDA and Spokane. It was constructed around the 1920's, and remained the primary highway until the 1960's when Interstate 90 was built. I-90 was routed along the northern edge of CDA. Highway 10 was a four-lane road with quite a bit of right-of-way on the north and south sides. When I-90 was opened, the Federal Highway Administration, and respective transportation departments from each state assumed responsibility of the new interstate system. Old highways were transferred to local jurisdictions. In this case, part of Old Highway 10 went to the City of Coeur d'Alene, and the majority of it went to the Post Falls Highway District.

When the routing plans for the proposed trail were finalized, the trail organizers presented the plans to the three entities who would ultimately own the trail. Those entities included Kootenai County, City of Post Falls, and the City of Coeur d'Alene. All three had endorsed the project, and the route, in concept. The presentations to the two cities were televised, in addition the Coeur d'Alene Press and Spokesman Review had covered numerous stories on the progress of the trail project. Once the historic railroad bridge at the state line had been secured and the trail supporters were notified of the federal appropriation to help with trail construction, trail opponents began to take notice. A united effort to stop the trail route campaigned vigorously enough to halt the already approved federal funding.

The City of CDA owned and maintained the land, and right-of-way, in which the trail traveled through in that city. It was not the same for the City of Post Falls, and Kootenai County. Post Falls had several county roads traversing through the city. Kootenai County did not maintain any roads. The county roads were managed and maintained by the Post Falls Highway District (PFHD). In an initial meeting with the Highway District in early 1988, the routing was identified, and their approval was sought for the trail to cross, or be on roads within their jurisdiction. The three PFHD Commissioners implied in that initial meeting that the trail project looked good to them. They would consider the routing, consult with their engineer, and get back to us.

The State of Idaho is comprised of multiple highway districts throughout the state. Each district is an independent government entity with authority to tax the residents in a given district for the long-term care and maintenance of the roads. The districts have elected officials representing a defined area. They have complete authority and final say over the management of the roadways. Overlapping of jurisdictions is common near cities and counties. The respective agencies do their best to communicate with one another to ensure safe roads. The focus of highway districts, for the most part, is on the movement of vehicles through their jurisdictions, not pedestrians.

A great deal of debate emerged from that initial meeting. Trail supporters, perhaps overly enthusiastic, believed the Highway District Commissioners were supporting the trail route. They stated as such in their reports to other entities, including our congressional representatives. Surprisingly, the PFHD took a position to prohibit the trail from using Seltice Way, citing safety issues and lack of planning on the part of the trail group. Their opposition to the trail route being on Seltice Way was supported by two lumber mills; Idaho Forest Industries, W-I Forest Products, and Central Pre-Mix Concrete Company. The lumber mills and concrete company considered it to be too risky to mix logging trucks and cement mixers with pedestrians and bicyclists on this corridor.

The City of Coeur d'Alene's jurisdiction, at that time, extended as far as Old Atlas Road on Seltice Way. Old Atlas Road was the western boundary of the city's area of impact, and about ¼ mile west of the current Atlas Road. West of Old Atlas Road, the Seltice Way corridor was in the jurisdiction of the PFHD, and it continued west all the way to the Idaho/Washington state line. Both lumber mills and the concrete company were along the roadways owned and maintained by the City of Coeur d'Alene, however, they were not part of the city. Their property and operations were located in the county, and had not been annexed into the city.

The PFHD Commissioners agreed with these concerns and decided they could not risk such liability on their road. When it became apparent that the Highway District now, suddenly would take a position to deny pedestrian and bicycle use of a public road, trail organizers requested additional meetings with them to identify, and possibly mitigate the concerns raised by the PFHD.

At one PFHD Board meeting in April of 1989, Coeur d'Alene City Councilman, Steve McCrae, attended the meeting to offer input and support. It was explained to the Highway commissioners that the concept of sharing a road was not new, or unique. There were many roadways with heavier use where cars and commercial activity exist with little, or no conflict. Seltice Way was not any different from those, and had plenty of right-of-way to allow for the construction of a trail separated from traffic. The highway commissioners maintained that they could not subject the district to the liability that would result from this proposed trail. Councilman McCrae asked the highway commissioners if their concern about liability could be absolved, would they support the trail route. The commissioners did not say yes or no, but stated they would consider it.

The liability debate continued for the better part of the year. While this discussion remained a priority topic, the PFHD Board of Commissioners were being lobbied by residents of the Pinevilla neighborhood and the commercial businesses along Seltice Way to deny the trail access on this road. Petitions and letters were submitted to the Highway District encouraging the denial of trail use anywhere near Seltice Way.

The idea of absolving the Highway District of liability was passed on to the Kootenai County Board of Commissioners for a legal opinion in May of 1989. The county prosecutor's office was asked to render an opinion on this discussion. The topic of absolving the PFHD of liability continued through most of the year.

On June 23, Carl Martin from Idaho Forest Industries sent letters to the Post Falls Highway District and the trail organizers, respectively, and sent copies to Senator McClure, Representative Craig, County Commissioners and the city councils of Post Falls and Coeur d'Alene. In his letter, Mr. Martin implored the PFHD to stop the trail project.

On June 27, 1989, PFHD Commissioner, Bob Wilbur sent a letter to Senator McClure, and may have summed up the viewpoint of trail opposers; Bob wrote, "We, in Kootenai County, have done without this proposed trail for a long time, hold up the funding, and give all the people of Kootenai County the true picture, the impact, environmental problems, and safety problems".

The debate on the routing of the trail raged on through most of 1989. On July 2, 1989 the Coeur d'Alene Press reported that Post Falls resident, Ned Zenger, had submitted nearly 300 signatures to the Post Falls City Council. The council had approved the routing, but were being accused of keeping information to themselves on the trail routing, and project. Mr. Zenger went on to say that the residents were not necessarily opposed to the trail, they just did not want it near their neighborhood and it was not safe for children. In the same article, Post Falls Highway Commissioner Bob Wilbur, was quoted as saying that he "would go to court to prevent the trail from being on Seltice Way".

July 14, 1989 Mr. Martin sent a second letter to the congressmen, PFHD, and Kootenai County Commissioners. This letter was more scathing and accused the trail planners of being untruthful and inaccurate.

On July 17, 1989, Kim Hansen, of W-I Forest Products, and a Pinevilla subdivision resident, also sent a letter to the Board of County Commissioners citing those 600 signatures had been collected opposing the trail location. This was also copied and sent to Senator McClure.

Letter writing from proponents and opponents occupied a considerable amount of time.

Trail opponents sent pages of letters to local jurisdictions and U.S. Congressmen stating that the trail process did not fully disclose alternative routes or identify hazards of the trail route presented to the public. Trail proponents responded with their own letters declaring that the trail opponents were uninformed and that due diligence was carefully and painstakingly evaluated along the entire corridor.

Trail opposers repeatedly said they were not opposed to the trail; they were just opposed to having it at this location . . . or that location . . . or that location . . . or that location. They did however, agree to the trail route being moved far north of Post Falls and Coeur d'Alene where it would be relatively inaccessible, unsafe, and very costly. Hmmm.

Finally, the county prosecutor's office rendered an opinion in October of 1989. *The Highway District already had a high degree of liability, and had not taken prudent steps to assure safe travels for all users. Pedestrians, runners, and bicyclists were at present using Seltice Way; and had been using it long before the proposal of the trail project began. Constructing a designated pedestrian pathway might actually reduce their liability. However, the Highway District cannot be absolved of meeting safety needs, nor absolved of liability.*

It was assumed that the highway district would acknowledge this legal opinion and work with the trail group to construct a safe route. Surprisingly, they did not. They doubled down saying there were alternative routes north of Seltice Way, and felt that the trail planners were negligent in identifying them in their routing plans. The two alternative routes that they wanted to be considered were Poleline Road and/or Prairie Avenue. Both were two lane roads going east and west. Those alternative routes were also in the

PFHD jurisdiction, and they implied that they would authorize trail use on either of those alternative routes.

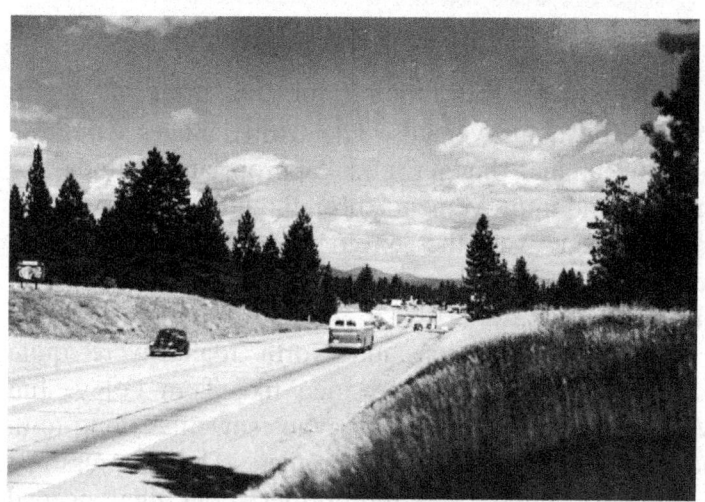

Photo Courtesy of North Idaho Museum

Highway 10 was the main, and only, east-west highway that went through North Idaho. It was a direct route to Spokane and beyond. This photo was taken in the 1950's. The new Interstate 90 was constructed in the 1960's, and shortly after that Highway 10 was renamed to Seltice Way.

Chapter 9
Federal Appropriation Halted

Securing federal funding for this project was, in itself, a bit controversial. The United States Congress sets an annual budget and 'appropriates' funds for projects and improvements throughout the country. This trail project was the only time these funds were requested, approved and issued for a local recreation project.

Eastern Washington and North Idaho were quite fortunate they had congressmen like Tom Foley, Jim McClure and Larry Craig who saw the long-term benefits of this bi-state trail project. The congressmen wanted to support the trail project, but they needed strong reasons to do so. Trail master plans from Idaho and Washington, along with financial plans, gave them reason to support the trail.

A contingency of people in the community did not believe the government should be making such appropriations, and believed it wrong for us to accept the funds.

Another contingency of people believed if the government was making such appropriations, North Idahoans should be requesting more of those funds to help get projects done that may otherwise not get funded. The Centennial Trail project was a good example for this line of thinking. The federal funds were going to be distributed regardless of our differences on the subject. Rather than see those funds go to Arizona, California, West Virginia, or any other state, trail supporters would say that the funds might as well be appropriated to Idaho and Washington.

The Post Falls Highway District did not wait for the county prosecutor's office to submit an opinion on PFHD's responsibility to provide safe routes for all users. The PFHD had already decided that this trail project would not be allowed on the Seltice Way corridor.

On June 27, 1989 the Highway Commissioners sent a letter to the Chairman of the federal appropriations committee, Senator Jim McClure, requesting that the *federal funds be frozen and the trail not be allowed to be built because right-of-ways, and routing was not properly secured, and the trail organizers did not do due diligence when planning this unsafe routing project.*

The PFHD also informed the Senator that *petitions had been signed by residents in Post Falls and businesses along the proposed route stating that they were adamantly opposed to the trail being located on Seltice Way.*

On June 28, 1989 the PFHD Board of Commissioners sent a letter to the Kootenai County Board of Commissioners, stating that the highway district *will not endorse the trail route on Seltice Way.* The letter further stated *the county commissioners did not give proper public notice to everyone impacted by the trail route.* This was a bit unfair towards the county commissioners. They entrusted the trail committee to plan and organize meetings. One county commissioner would take the PFHD to task over their comments.

Senator McClure contacted me as chairman for the trail project, requesting to stop progress on the trail until this matter could be resolved. The senator expressed his surprise this issue had come up after the funding appropriation had been approved. He believed the routing for the trail had been secured thus implying he had been misled by the trail organizers. Senator

THE TRAIL THAT ALMOST WASN'T

McClure's request to stop the trail development stunned the trail organizers.

The federal appropriation that was budgeted for the North Idaho Centennial Trail was not administered locally. The administration of the funding became the responsibility of the U.S. Forest Service in Missoula, Montana. That office also requested that the trail committee place a temporary hold on spending the federal funds. The Missoula office explained that the appropriation is earmarked for the North Idaho Centennial Trail and stopping development does not have to occur as long as the funds are being used for the trail. The senator can request that the project stop until the PFHD issue is resolved. However, it is only a request and does not have to be adhered to.

Kootenai County was the lead sponsor for the trail project regarding the federal appropriation. The funds are authorized for a specific project and Kootenai County accepted the duty of financial oversight. The county was responsible for awarding contracts for trail development and submitting payment to the forest service who would, in turn, authorize reimbursement from the federal government. After the county commissioners were apprised of the senator's request, and out of respect for the senator, they rightfully complied with his request to halt the project until the routing issues were resolved. Senator McClure, unlike Governor Andrus, and Representative Craig, did not have the opportunity to tour the proposed routing of the trail.

Tension continued between the county, the trail organizers and the PFHD. On July 7, 1989, County Commissioner Evalyn Adams responded to Senator McClure's request and to the Post Falls Highway District commissioners. She explained the concerns raised by the PFHD had been addressed throughout the planning stages in 1988, including public meetings and alternative routing. The trail debate escalated as the county commissioner admonished the PFHD for creating false allegations concerning the trail planning, and the process.

Chapter 10
The Death of the Trail

The controversy on Seltice Way, Old Highway 10, was taking a serious toll on the fund-raising efforts to build the trail. On August 4th, 1989, the Adjutant Group resigned as the trail's premiere fund raiser. Adjutant said that *fighting well-organized opposition is just too time consuming. In reality, the trail faces an uphill battle, which has been precipitated by a few shrewd businessmen, and one (Post Falls) highway district official, who is functioning in the definitive conflict of interest.*

Post Falls Highway District Commissioner, Bob Wilbur, owned a business on Seltice Way. His business was at the mid-way point of the proposed route on Seltice Way. Many trail supporters believed the commissioner should have recused himself on the trail routing decisions. Two days prior to Adjutant's resigning, the Post Falls Highway District Board of Commissioners voted unanimously to deny the North Idaho Centennial Trail access to Seltice Way. This vote, combined with Adjutant's resignation, created a giant setback in the trail planning and development. Trail committee member and Kootenai County Commissioner, Evalyn Adams, said, "Their act (PFHD) was certainly unexpected, and could mean the death of the trail."

The Post Falls Highway District voted to not allow the trail to be located from the 1600 block to the 2500 block on Seltice Way. The PFHD office is located near the middle of this section that they were banning the trail supporters from using. The 1600 block began in Post Falls where the Tidyman's grocery store was located, today it is Yokes grocery store. Tidyman's was a big sponsor of the trail and was not in opposition to the trail location on Seltice Way. The ban extended into Coeur d'Alene to the east side of Central Pre-Mix. Today that area is the entrance into the Riverstone Subdivision off of Seltice Way.

Fundraising took a huge set back. Coupling this with letters sent to Senator McClure by the PFHD to stop the funding of the trail placed the trail in limbo. Senator McClure, having received letters indicating the trail route was pre-maturely planned and approved without local jurisdiction authority, requested a halt to the use of the funds. Senator McClure reiterated that he did not want to see the trail built in sporadic sections, leaving some sections undone due to routing conflicts.

A war of words escalated from the action of the PFHD.

On August 5, 1989 a dedication ceremony was held in the Coeur d'Alene City Park. The CDA City Council had already dedicated the trail route through the city, and the city route ran along the sea wall through the park.

The Panhandle Kiwanis Club was involved in various civic projects and had offered to add new benches, trees, and improve the concrete walkway along the designated route through the City Park. Club President, Mike Boyd, in his dedication speech said, "With the recent hold on federal funds until the route is finalized, and the Post Falls Highway District commissioner's decision that the route cannot use Seltice Way, this project is in *extreme jeopardy.*"

Chapter 11
The Lumber Mills

Dating back to the late 1800's, timber harvesting was a major industry in this part of the country. Several lumber entrepreneurs, such as Frederick Blackwell, D. C. Corbin and others, invested heavily in the transportation of trees to the lumber mills for processing into building materials. Coeur d'Alene Lake and the Spokane River were ideal transportation routes for the harvested trees. The trees would be cut in the nearby forests, hauled to the lake and corralled in large log booms that could contain hundreds of logs. The booms could be moved across the lake and down the river by tug boats. This process continued well into the 1990's. Several pilings, which helped to hold the logs once they reached their mill destination along the river, can still be seen in some places. This was a very sizable industry in Kootenai County for nearly a century and employed thousands that were connected to the timber industry.

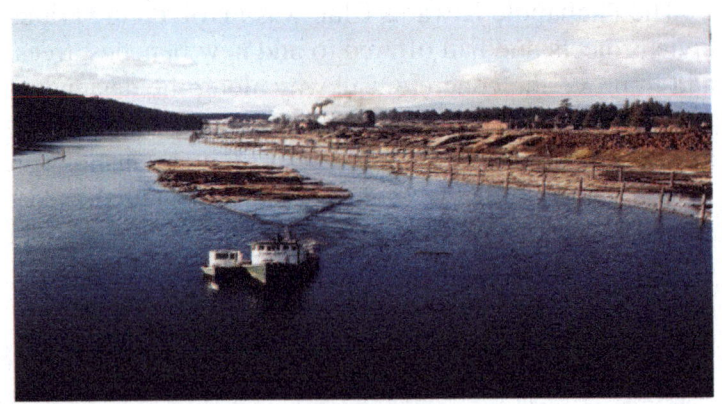

Photo Courtesy of North Idaho Museum

Logging was a major industry in North Idaho for many decades. Trucks would bring logs to the lumber mills from the highway, and tug boats would two large log booms across the lake and down the river to the mills. This photo depicts the logs being towed to the IFI and W-I Forest Products sites along the Spokane River. Seltice Way/Old Highway 10 is to the right of the photo, not visible.

Logging and cement mixer trucks were a common sight throughout North Idaho, and even more prevalent on Seltice Way. Seven lumber mills operated in the immediate area between Coeur d'Alene and Post Falls. Two of them were on the proposed routing for the Centennial Trail, causing concerns with over-sized trucks possibly interacting with pedestrians. Two lumber mills; W-I Forest Products and Idaho Forest Industries were both located on Seltice Way along the roadway controlled by the City of Coeur d'Alene. Sharing the road was not an option from the standpoint of the mill managers. The lumber mills opposed the trail route and lobbied the Post Falls Highway District to deny access for such a trail. The mills also cited liability, safety and lack of planning by the trail organizers. The trail organizers met with the mill managers on several occasions in an attempt to find common ground for the trail and the trucks. That common ground was not to be found.

W-I Forest Products, an Oregon based company, sent representative Kim Hanson to attend the meetings. Kim was also a resident of the Pinevilla neighborhood where hundreds of signatures were gathered on a petition opposing the trail route. The trail routing issue was at its peak of debate through most of 1989. At one meeting with W-I Forest Products, trail organizers questioned why the mill was so opposed to the trail. The response was reiterated, "It is not safe and not responsible."

THE TRAIL THAT ALMOST WASN'T

Co-chair of the trail committee, Randy Haddock stated he *heard W-I Forest Products intended to close the mill. If that happened then there would be no issue with the trail route.* W-I Forrest Products strongly denied rumors of the mill closing.

Shortly after that meeting, in May of 1990, W-I Forest Products did indeed announce that the mill was closing and laying off 130 mill workers. This was the second mill closing announcement. Potlatch Forest Products (Rutledge Mill) located on the east end of Coeur d'Alene announced their closing earlier in 1987. Logging practices were changing, and within the next 15 years, the once flourishing timber industry would completely disappear from the northern shoreline of Lake Coeur d'Alene and along the Spokane River.

For the time being, the mill position remained in a no-compromise position for a mix of uses with regard to a pedestrian trail. Idaho Forest Industries (IFI) used a truck scale on their property that would sometimes create a long line of logging trucks waiting to be weighed at that mill site. Those trucks would be queued along the south side of Seltice Way.

IFI was also involved in the community on many different levels. They were the most participatory mill in the area with regards to the community, and community enhancements. The mill and the city enjoyed an effective working relationship. The Coeur d'Alene Parks Department frequently called upon IFI over the years for assistance with several different park projects. Tom Richards, the owner of IFI, was well-known for his involvement in the community. The IFI administrative staff gathered together local mills for donations when the Coeur d'Alene Parks Department was building the Rotary Lakeside Bandshell in the Coeur d'Alene City Park. Nearly all of the lumber materials were donated for that project. IFI also contributed to nearly every playground in the city parks system by supplying the surface material placed beneath the playground structures. However, the Centennial Trail project tested that relationship to its very limits.

The Coeur d'Alene City Council was not budging from their position to support the proposed routing of the trail along Northwest Boulevard and Seltice Way in the Coeur d'Alene City limits. The council maintained that the commercial trucking and vehicle traffic could be compatible with a designated pedestrian trail. The mill site administration would not accept this point of view. From the mills' point of view, it was simply too dangerous to mix big rigs with pedestrians and bicycles. The mills were especially concerned with the trail passing in front of their operation where the big trucks had to access the mill site.

The mills continued to insist that the Post Falls Highway District deny trail access onto Seltice Way. If the Highway District would not give permission to use Seltice Way then the proposed trail would be at a dead end, which they thought would be unacceptable per the terms of the federal appropriation. The trail had to be continuous with no breaks in the routing. A discontinuance in the trail routing would force the trail organizers to re-route the trail north of Coeur d'Alene and Post Falls, or abandon the project.

The issue being raised by the Post Falls Highway District was that of liability. The City of Coeur d'Alene, City of Post Falls and Kootenai County stood firm that Seltice Way continued to be the corridor of choice, and the liability issues could be mitigated. The PFHD had expressed they would not support the route and would take the issue to court to deny the trail from having access onto Seltice Way. Trail proponents and opponents were polarized over this trail idea, and neither side was willing to back down.

Another informational meeting, hosted by the Kootenai County Commissioners, was held at North Idaho College on August 10, 1989. With approximately 300 people attending, the crowd was about equally divided between proponents and opponents regarding trail issues. The meeting was contentious and the next day the Press reported that the Coeur d'Alene Chamber of Commerce suggested a 30-day cooling off period. That did not happen.

Making matters worse, long-time trail supporter and county commissioner, Evalyn Adams, resigned from the trail committee the day after this meeting. In her words, she felt 'flayed' at the public meeting. She went on to say that she cannot communicate with the PFHD effectively and that her credibility with U.S. Senator McClure had been tainted as a result of the comments made about her. She believed it to be in the best interest of the trail project if she excused her-self from further active participation. The trail committee, in a show of support, voted to not accept her resignation. She expressed her appreciation of the committee but reiterated that she would be stepping down from the committee effective immediately.

The commissioner's resignation from the trail committee came one week after the resignation of the fund-raising efforts of the Adjutant Group. The darkest days of the trail project could be said to be those of the summer of 1989. Fund raising had all but stopped, a major trail advocate was leaving the committee and trail opponents were gathering signatures by the 100's to stop, or relocate the trail. In spite of major setbacks, trail proponents kept moving forward.

Ray Stone, mayor of Coeur d'Alene, was called upon by the opposition to rethink the routing and relocate the trail. Mayor Stone stood by the routing and did not acquiesce. 1989 was an election year. Some interest grew within the group of trail opponents to bring in a challenger to unseat the mayor, who would support relocating the trail away from the Seltice corridor.

In September 1989 it was rumored through Huckleberries, a weekly column in the Spokesman Review, that Tom Richards of IFI was entertaining an idea to have someone run against the CDA mayor.

On October 4th, 1989, Lee Shellman, former chairman of the state Republican Party announced he was conducting a poll to gauge support for his run at the mayor's seat.

On October 5th, he announced the poll results were good and that he would make a decision soon. The decision to enter the mayoral race against incumbent Mayor Stone never came. Later however, Lee Shellman volunteered to be on the Coeur d'Alene Parks & Recreation Commission and became a staunch supporter of all thing's parks and trails.

On November 7th, at a Chamber of Commerce banquet, Tom Richards, owner and founder of IFI, was recognized for the Distinguished Citizen of the Year Award. He was asked about his support to have Lee Shellman run for CDA Mayor. Tom said, "I was actually supporting Bandito (his dog) to run, but the canine was not talking about it." Tom was very successful in the timber industry, a huge supporter of the community, and he maintained a good sense of humor.

The following year, 1990, another canine would be front and center, on a different trail issue near the terminus of the proposed 23-mile trail.

Chapter 12
Where There is Smoke . . .

Two burning issues heated up residents of Kootenai County for most of the 1980's, especially the latter part...*grass burning* and *the Centennial Trail*. Like the lumber mills, bluegrass growing and seed harvesting became a significant industry in the area. Kentucky Bluegrass was the choice for most growers and homeowners for its color, texture, and durability. Across most of the Northern United States, bluegrass is one of the best cool season ground covers. Thousands and thousands of acres throughout the Rathdrum Prairie, and the Palouse were bluegrass fields.

One of the largest growers in the area was Jacklin Seed. They sold seed products throughout many parts of the world. The most controversial part of that industry was the controlled field burning which occurred every fall. The burning usually did not last longer than a two-week period. The planned burns increased the seed productivity. Several studies were done to determine a better way to enhance the seed production, but nothing did the job as well as burning.

While the field burning issues were being addressed, the Post Falls Highway District was dealing with an issue of their own. That issue had to do with what people perceived as a negative impact on their quality of life, their health, and on the environment. The PFHD was operating a rock crushing quarry on Prairie Avenue just west of Highway 41. Residents in the area were complaining of the dust and noise contributed by the rock crushing operation.

The quarry was in Kootenai County, and the nearby residents called upon the county to step in and regulate the operation, and/or have it relocated to a more rural area. The complaints registered with the county stated that the rock crushing equipment was operated 24 hours a day, seven days a week, without end. After a continuous two-week period of non-stop crushing, and a non-sympathetic response from the highway district, the residents sought legal counsel.

The nexus between grass burning, rock crushing, and Centennial Trail routing was apparent, albeit frustrating, to the trail committee. Grass field burning as well as the rock crushing operation posed real health problems. Both were located on one of the very same roadways in which the Post Falls Highway District demanded that the trail be located: Prairie Avenue. Bluegrass farms were along Prairie Ave. and Poleline Ave., which would have placed bicyclists, runners, walkers and children directly into the center of the smoke and dust. The health issues alone were enough to avoid such a location for a pedestrian trail. Visibility during seasonal field burnings was reduced to a minimum, compounding the health and safety of pedestrians.

The large number of acres burned caused a significant amount of smoke in the air. The smoke had a negative impact on tourism as well as on people's health. The practice of field burning had gone on for decades, but as the community grew in population, and the mining and timber industries began to give way to the hospitality industry, field burning was becoming a greater issue.

The smoke from the fields would hover over the community, causing breathing problems for people with allergies, or asthma, and the smoke obscured the incredible scenery that people wanted to see and enjoy. Grass burning would typically begin in early September as students were returning to school. Demonstrators would gather in front of the Jacklin Seed office to protest. They petitioned the Governor and state legislators to 'Stop Field Burning.' The opposition to field burning went beyond Kootenai County and included Spokane and Nez Perce Counties, Worley, and the Columbia Basin.

The Idaho Division of Environmental Quality blamed field burning for the worst smoke days of the year. The CDA Press reported that more than 100 calls *per day* were logged at the DEQ office during the field burning season. Environmental, tourism, and health issues stayed at the forefront, with some people being hospitalized and others being forced to use a respirator during the days of field burning. Elderly people, and the very young, seemed to be hit the hardest. Dr. Mayer Horensten D.O., admitted some of his patients to Kootenai Medical Center (now Kootenai Health) stating, *"People were not critically ill from the grass burning, but they were miserable because of it."* A class-action law suit eventually brought a phased-out end to the grass burning.

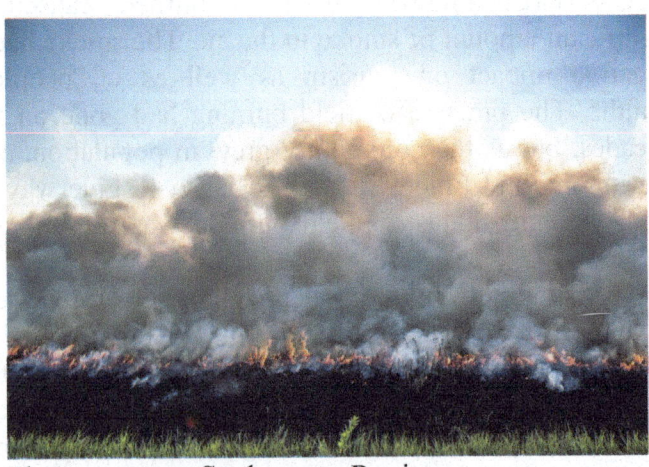

Photo courtesy Spokesman Review

For the trail planners, the situation came down to these two facts. One: The concerns of the mills and PFHD that logging trucks or cement mixers could not co-exist in an area that had enough right of way to allow for a separated pedestrian trail, was not a reasonable position. Two: The alternative, which was soundly rejected by the trail planners, was to recommend that pedestrians be sent into an identified health, and environmentally unsafe area.

The trail committee and its supporters were unwavering in their belief that Seltice Way was the best location for the trail. The PFHD was equally adamant that they would not allow the trail on Seltice Way. The threat by the highway district to take the issue to court was welcomed by the trail supporters. They looked forward to presenting their case to a district Judge for a ruling regarding a safe route for pedestrians, and if pedestrians and bicyclists could, in fact, be denied access to a public road that *they were already using*. Until that could happen, problems continued to mount for the trail committee. The project continued to sit with funds being frozen and fund-raising slowing to a trickle.

A two mile stretch of trail, nearly in the middle of the proposed 23-mile trail system would hold up everything and possibly result in the demise of the entire trail.

Chapter 13
A Disconnected Trail

Although the City of Post Falls had approved the trail routing through their community, it remained uncertain how the trail would connect to the City of Coeur d'Alene. Rather than proceed with trail development to the west of Spokane Street, it was decided to wait and see how things played out with the issues involving the Highway District, especially in the event a judge ruled against the trail routing.

The City of Coeur d'Alene held steadfast to the idea of approval for the original trail route. They allowed for the design documents to be prepared so the trail could be further developed when the issues were resolved. The trail on the east side of Seltice Way would connect to Northwest Boulevard. This section of Northwest Boulevard was part of the I-90 Business Loop. Northwest Boulevard was a four-lane road with little room at that time to install a separated trail from vehicle traffic.

The trail routing along this boulevard would have a 3-foot class II trail on the river side of the road. A wider area for the trail could not be created due to the needed width of the vehicle lanes; four lanes with a fifth lane for left hand turns. This would be the least desirable section of the trail for a length of one mile. It remained that way until the mills closed, and the land was bought by a developer, John Stone. He granted access for the trail through the Riverstone subdivision in 2006. This brought great happiness to the North Idaho Centennial Trail Foundation members and the City of Coeur d'Alene.

The trail veered off of Northwest Boulevard, southward at Lincoln Way, near the North Idaho College campus and traveled along Rosenberry Drive, which became West Lakeshore Drive, until it reached the Coeur d'Alene City Park. All the controversy swirling around the trail did not seem to affect the people in Coeur d'Alene. They were increasingly supportive of the trail and its routing.

The Boy Scouts of America (BSA) owned a ½ acre parcel of land that was directly between the trail and the lake along West Lakeshore Drive. BSA made this land a gift deed to the Coeur d'Alene Parks Department in October of 1992, enabling trail users to have the opportunity for waterfront access from the Centennial Trail.

Another resident along West Lakeshore Drive, Terry Porcerelli, supported the trail route, which passed directly in front of her home. She noticed a dead Ponderosa Pine tree on the recently gifted land and called the CDA Parks Office with a request that her brother, who dabbled in chain saw artwork, cut a bench from the large dead tree stump for people to sit and admire the lake while using the Centennial Trail. The offer to volunteer her brother was well received, and he sculpted a chair-seat out of the tree stump. Even though the spirits of the trail committee were being pushed down with the unexpected and unfounded opposition, this type of support lifted their spirits.

The trail split in two directions when it reached the City Park. The pedestrians were routed along the seawall, while bicyclists were routed along the northern part of the park. Pedestrian traffic, in the Coeur d'Alene City Park and along the sea wall, remained very busy during the summer months. Routing bicycles around the pedestrian crowds proved to be easy and safe. The pedestrian and bicycle sections reconnected at Independence Point, flowing eastward past the CDA Resort and through the northern edge of McEuen Park. It continued along Mullan Avenue to the eastern boundary of the city limits at Lake Coeur d'Alene Drive.

This was the point where the old Interstate 90 was being relocated, and the trail committee had anticipated picking up one of the abandoned four lanes to carry the trail five miles beyond Coeur d'Alene to Higgins Point.

For the time being, routing had been approved through most of Post Falls, awaiting the outcome of the PFHD issues on Seltice Way. Routing was also approved through Coeur d'Alene. Construction plans were being developed, but the trail could not be built until the Seltice Way issue was resolved. The frustration of waiting grew intense.

Chapter 14
Seltice Way and Interstate 90

The tumultuous issues over the use of Seltice Way were far reaching. A plethora of meetings occurred with proponents, opponents, and third parties who took a neutral position. One of those neutral parties was the District 1 Office of the Idaho Transportation Department, led by District Engineer Scott Stokes.

Scott unexpectedly stopped by the CDA Parks Office in 1990. He said he was aware of the controversy regarding the routing of the Centennial Trail through the industrial corridor on Seltice Way. He suggested, as an alternative and temporary solution, that the trail committee consider using the south side of the Interstate right-of-way, between Northwest Boulevard in Coeur d'Alene, and Highway 41 in Post Falls. Trail planners had not given that option any consideration during the planning process. Pedestrian and bicycle use within an Interstate right-of-way were not common. Transportation departments, almost exclusively deny that type of mixed use in their right-of-way. The difference here is when Interstate 90 was developed through North Idaho in the 1960's, the Federal Highway Administration and the Idaho Department of Transportation acquired a wide section of land for the four-lane interstate and for possible expansion in the future.

Trail designer, Jon Mueller and I walked the right-of-way to see if this could be a possible solution. The south side of the Interstate right-of-way happened to be the highest ground in the Interstate corridor. It also had quite a few mature Ponderosa Pine trees growing in the right-of-way. It was suggested that the trail could

THE TRAIL THAT ALMOST WASN'T

meander through the Ponderosa Pines. The trail distance from the I-90 travel lanes, and its elevation above the Interstate would not create a risk factor for trail users.

ITD was contacted and informed that this could be a viable solution to the current stand-off between the Highway District and the municipalities. In response, the trail committee was directed to seek approval from the ITD Board. If Consent was granted, the trail routing would have support from the ITD District I office.

Plans were drawn up with oversight of the ITD Engineers to assure that the trail would not pose any conflicts within the transportation corridor, including erosion of the embankment. The trail committee, the county, and the municipalities were made aware that if this route were to be approved, it would probably only be a temporary route. The trail would have to be maintained by Kootenai County and the cities as long as it remained in the ITD right-of-way. The temporary status of the route was due to the fact that should the Interstate need to be expanded, the trail would be removed from the right-of-way. A state and local agreement would be drafted if the Transportation Board allowed use of the right-of-way, so their successors, and trail successors, would not have issues over this temporary use.

Although this appeared to be a solution to the Seltice Way issues, a few problems popped up that could lead to trail development costs prohibiting the use of this corridor. Major problems involved crossing two roads; Atlas Road in Coeur d'Alene and Huetter Road in the county. Those two roads would have to be bridged, creating a major cost increase.

When ITD became aware that the cost of building two bridges may prohibit the trail from being built in their right-of-way, ITD stepped up again. They had a couple of construction projects in other parts of the state where two bridges were being removed and those bridges could work well for the purposes of the trail. The trail group had to incur the cost of transporting, installing, and refurbishing the bridges, which was more cost effective than constructing new bridges.

An official request to use the right-of-way was presented to the Transportation Board in late 1990. The request to use the Interstate right-of-way was approved the following year, with the condition that the trail be maintained by the municipalities. The design and construction would need to meet the standards and requirements of ITD. A second fence would need to be installed between the trail and the Interstate. A fence would be on the north and south sides of the trail. This was to prevent pedestrians from wandering too close to the Interstate. All parties involved in the battle over Seltice Way got on board and endorsed this alternative, temporary route. A major conflict was finally averted and the Idaho Transportation Department became the hero of the day.

Chapter 15
Slip Slidin' Away...

In 1987, during the early days in the design planning stages, the trail committee had their eye on the soon-to-be abandoned section of the Interstate east of Coeur d'Alene. Their goal was to secure the lakeside lane of the 4-lane highway. This would complete the final 5 miles of the Centennial Trail. Before the trail committee began talking about this section, there was already interest in improving this area for outdoor recreation.

Jack Roos, a retired engineer from the Idaho Transportation Department, and Rick Cummins, District 1 Superintendent for the north region of the Idaho Department of Parks and Recreation, made a 'pitch' to the Four Northern Counties Natural Resources Committee. They told the Natural Resources Committee that there may be an opportunity to expand the boat launch parking lot near Higgins Point, improve the boat launch, and add a pedestrian/bicycle route along one of the four abandoned Interstate lanes. The Natural Resources Committee, led by Sandy Emerson, endorsed the idea and forwarded it on to the Kootenai County Commissioners for their endorsement.

This particular section of the proposed trail route was in the county, just east of the Coeur d'Alene city limits. One of the County Commissioners had been an active participant with the trail planning committee, and was very supportive of this future opportunity. ITD was made aware of the desire by the county to enhance this whole five-mile stretch for public outdoor recreation, however ITD was not interested in doing that.

They (ITD) had already planned to make some parking lot improvements at the boat launch area near

Higgins Point as part of the Interstate relocation. The parking lot improvements were immediately adjacent to a new Interstate on-ramp that was proposed as part of the new highway project. ITD was hopeful that they would transfer the old highway to the Eastside Highway District once the new Interstate was opened. Neither ITD nor the East Side Highway District was interested in a pedestrian/bicycle trail adjacent to vehicle traffic. Both entities were in the business of moving vehicles, not pedestrians, and they expressed no interest in public outdoor recreation. Extending the trail east of Coeur d'Alene to Higgins Point looked like a pipe dream that would not become a reality.

It was early 1990 (March 28th,) when a section of the soon-to-be-abandoned Interstate 90 slid into the lake. The area is where fill material was being brought in to expand the roadway for the creation of a new on-ramp. The ITD contractor had brought in 650,000 cubic yards of fill material, which was not stable enough to support the roadway as intended. The collapse of the embankment took part of the highway and caused traffic delays along the I-90 route since the new relocated I-90 had not yet been opened.

Compounding the problem of the new roadway and on-ramp, there was a threat of a pending strike that would hold up the I-90 relocation project. In April of 1990, the Teamsters Union General Local 690 notified ITD that they intended to strike against the Interstate project. The issue was that the general contractor, Scarcella Brothers of Seattle, who had hired workers mostly from the Seattle area instead of workers from the Spokane area. The construction project was in Idaho, and Idaho has a *right-to-work law*, which became part of the rumored strike issue.

On May 18, 1990, disaster struck again. Another larger area slipped into the lake, taking with it two multi-ton earth moving pieces of equipment; a bulldozer and a scraper. A father and son were operating the equipment as the slide occurred, and they rode the equipment right into the lake. Both operators escaped serious injury. This second slide led to a dispute between the general contractor and ITD over the fill material being used.

A scuba diver was dispatched the next day to locate the equipment which was thought to be about 100 feet below the surface of water, located just east of the current boat launch. The equipment was found, but it had been buried with the slide material, and only the vertical exhaust pipes were visible above the fill material. Several attempts were made to pull the equipment out of the lake, but every attempt failed.

On May 21, 1990, the Kootenai Environmental Alliance (KEA) threatened to sue the Idaho Transportation Department over the loss of the lake that 650,000 cubic yards of fill material now occupied. Fuel and oil leakage from the equipment, as well as loss of Kokanee Spawning grounds as a result of the land slide, were also cited in the claim.

Local attorney Scott Reed represented KEA in this lawsuit. ITD responded to this threat stating that the fill material was sound. A soil specialist was called in to evaluate the issue and determined that the fill material being used by ITD was 'ok.' They were allowed to proceed with the highway construction.

Another environmental group, Save Our Shores, joined in the concern raised by KEA. The two groups again questioned the permitting of the fill material. The Army Corps of Engineers had jurisdiction over the waters. They responded to the issue by stating the permit specifically stated angular rock was to be used as fill material. It was determined that dirt was being added with the rock, raising stability questions.

Scott Reed, the attorney representing KEA, and planning to file the lawsuit against ITD, was an extraordinary individual. He was not only a brilliant and respected attorney, but also had quite a sense of humor. On May 30, 1990, Scott Reed set out to prove his theory that the fill material was in fact polluting the lake. His method, a classic Scott Reed tongue-in-cheek approach, was to bring an expert to the slide area and have it proven once and for all that the lake area was contaminated. Scott threw a stick out into the lake. The expert swam out to get it and upon returning to the shore, he was followed by a plume of debris. Scott considered the demonstration a success. The expert was none other than his faithful golden retriever, Pedro.

The situation along the old Interstate corridor continued to worsen for ITD. The general contractor contacted OSHA (Occupational Safety and Health Association) with concerns that the fill material was still unsafe to work upon. OSHA ordered the work stopped until further studies could be done. They ultimately barred any further work until a new method of dumping fill material and its distribution in the slide area could be implemented.

In late June of 1990, the Idaho Department of Fish and Game came out with a statement that the slide area had probably destroyed the Kokanee Salmon and Trout spawning beds. That was an unpleasant message to the fishermen, who became concerned about the future of fishing on Lake Coeur d'Alene, not to mention the survival of the fish for their own sake.

The U.S. Army Corps of Engineers cited the Scarcella Brothers construction company and the Idaho

Transportation Department for an unfinished drainage ditch in the construction area that rapidly eroded in the rainy season. Soon after that, OSHA fined the general contractor.

Idaho State Senator, Denny Davis, invited the departments of Idaho Fish and Game, Idaho Department of Lands, and the Department of Environmental Quality to a public meeting. The purpose was to address public concerns about the landslide and subsequent contamination.

Two months later work was allowed to resume on the highway construction site with a new method of moving the fill material about the site. A conveyor system would be used to haul the fill material from the trucks to the site instead of having trucks backing into the slide area.

The Scarcella Brothers filed a claim against ITD for the loss of the earth moving equipment that could not be recovered from the bottom of the lake. The claim was in the amount of $150,000. Workers at the construction site were reluctant to return to the slide area. When they did return, they wore life jackets while operating the earth moving equipment.

The problems with the new highway construction and on-ramp seemed to be insurmountable, and in August of 1990, ITD proposed to the Federal Highway Administration that the on-ramp construction be abandoned. This led to more public scrutiny, and whether or not the on-ramp was ever needed in the first place.

KEA, and Scott Reed, filed the lawsuit citing violations of the Clean Water Act and related federal and state laws. The lawsuit also demanded that the fill material, that had been dumped in the lake, be removed and that ITD start over. The lawsuit identified various areas in which ITD could mitigate the damage done by the slide, which included the acquisition of wetland areas and other sites that could be preserved as an environment for native animals. The development of the pedestrian bicycle trail and public outdoor recreation enhancements along the five-mile corridor were not mentioned as possible mitigation in the lawsuit.

The Idaho Attorney General (AG) also considered bringing suit against the Idaho Transportation Department. The AG cited that the permit obtained by ITD to do the work had expired. ITD obtained the permit in the early 1970's when they were in the planning stages for the I-90 relocation project. However, the permit was valid for only 5 years and had not been renewed. ITD refuted this claim by the AG.

By late 1990, state representatives, specifically from Northern Idaho, were calling upon ITD to extend the Centennial Trail along the corridor using the lakeside lane of the soon-to-be abandoned I-90. They were recommending a scenic 2-lane road with turnouts, fishing docks, improved parking, and boat launching facilities.

ITD agreed in 1991 to include public outdoor recreation facilities along the 5-mile corridor. Nearly two more years passed before plans were approved for the Centennial Trail to be constructed. Other improvements would occur at Higgins Point, a state-owned property that would become the terminus of the Centennial Trail.

The estimated cost of these improvements was 2.4 million dollars. ITD approved the budget amount, and work began on the trail east of Coeur d'Alene in 1994. One year later, July 27, 1995, the last section of the 23-mile North Idaho Centennial Trail was completed, nearly 9 years after the concept was introduced. Thousands of people became involved in this trail project over that period of time. The final cost of the 23-mile trail, from the Washington-Idaho state line to Higgins Point, was just under *five million dollars.*

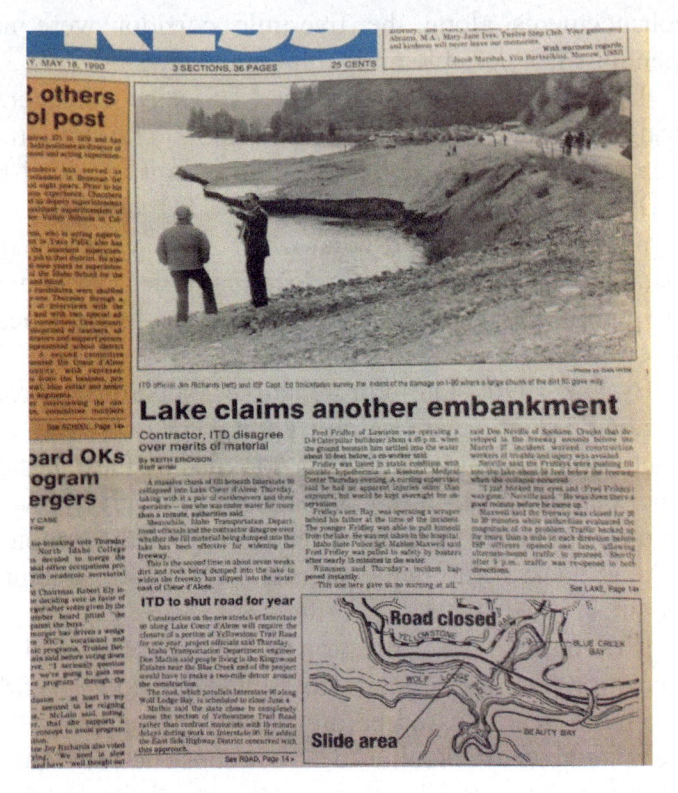

CDA Press, May 19, 1990

Engineers at the slide area near Higgens Point.

Chapter 16
Long-Term Problem Solving

Some areas along the trail route were considered problem areas by the trail committee. These areas were not ideal sections of the trail corridor due to vehicle traffic, street crossings and trail route identification.

Highway 41 and Seltice Way was one of the problem areas, commonly referred to as 'malfunction junction.' The confusing traffic signs and interstate access points led the public to giving it this adopted name. This intersection was also the connection point to the Centennial Trail along the interstate right-of-way. Trail routing along this right-of-way mitigated the issue between the trail committee and the PFHD on the use of Seltice Way. The sounds of vehicle horns were not uncommon when a driver steers into the wrong turn lane or hesitates too long because he/she is not certain of which lane they should be in.

This intersection was managed by the Idaho Transportation Department (ITD). Interstate on-ramps and off-ramps converge onto the intersection combined with multiple right and left-hand turn lanes, and a lot of interesting traffic signs.

Post Falls became the fastest growing city in Idaho and this intersection could not adequately support the volume of vehicles put upon it. A north bound state highway (Highway 41), east and west bound interstate on-ramps and off-ramps and east and west bound boulevard traffic all converge at this intersection.

The good news was that ITD was in the planning and design stages to re-build the intersection, including different locations for the interstate on-ramps and off-ramps. The reconstruction is targeted for 2025, including safe and easy passage for the Centennial Trail and its users.

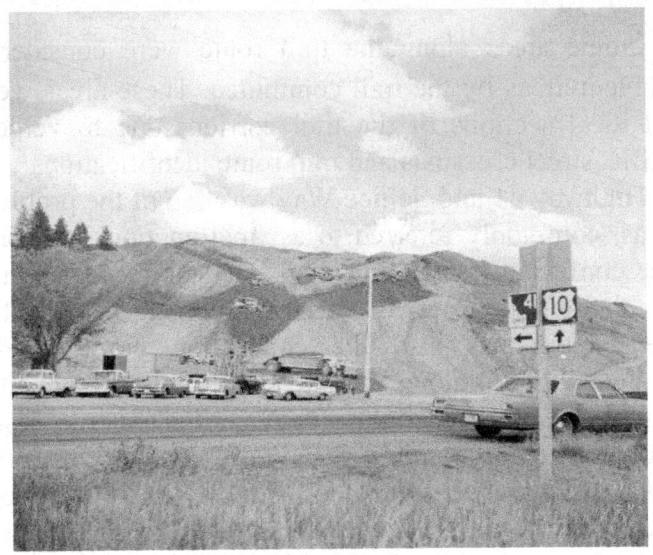

Photo courtesy of North Idaho Museum

The above photo was taken before Interstate 90 was completed in the early 1960's. This is the intersection of Highway 10 (Seltice Way) and Highway 41.

Northwest Boulevard in Coeur d'Alene was another problem area along the trail corridor. Its narrow class II trail was a temporary solution for the trail on this boulevard. Ten years had passed since the trail was built, and the goal to locate the trail closer to the river remained a high priority. In the early 2000s, Northwest Boulevard was scheduled to be rebuilt from the Interstate 90 interchange into downtown Coeur d'Alene; one mile in length. The Centennial Trail did not get included in the reconstruction process. This created a one-mile gap in the trail connectivity and caused concern among members of the trail foundation and trail users.

Developer John Stone had recently purchased the W-I Forest Products Mill site that bordered Northwest Boulevard. He was planning to build a live-work-play subdivision and offered to allow the trail to meander through this area bringing the trail closer to the Spokane River. A designated trail route along the river had not yet been identified. However, rumors were swirling that the railroad was considering abandoning their lines in that area.

Rebuilding Northwest Boulevard created other logistical issues for businesses along the corridor. A few of those businesses included the DeArmond Stud Mill near North Idaho College and Idaho Forest Industries on Seltice Way. They needed to haul lumber material from site to site and Northwest Boulevard was their business route.

Union Pacific Railroad (UP) and Burlington Northern Santa Fe Railroad (BNSF) serviced the mills. Their tracks were on Bureau of Land Management property which the railroads had leased from the U.S. Government for decades and decades. The mills were able to enter into an agreement with the railroad to allow for a 'haul road' to be built on the east side of the railroad tracks. This would be a temporary haul road for logging trucks to use until Northwest Boulevard was completed.

The trail foundation and the city requested to use the west side of the railroad right-of-way allowing the trail to connect the new Riverstone subdivision to downtown Coeur d'Alene. The railroads rejected that idea. They stated that pedestrians and bicycles in close proximity to trains would be too dangerous. The BLM, however, supported the idea as it fit their definition of public outdoor recreation on BLM property.

The Trail organizers had been recipients of several rejections over the course of building the Centennial Trail. This most recent one was disappointing but it would not be a deterrent. The movement that had begun in the 1980's to convert rails to trails was witnessing another ideology; *'rails with trails'*. This movement had merit, and it was being accomplished in other areas of the country. After months of discussion, the railroads acquiesced and agreed to allow the trail in the rail corridor with conditions. The foremost condition was that the trail must be physically separated from the train tracks. This could be accomplished by installing a four-foot-high chain link fence along the nearly one mile of the railroad right-of-way.

The relocation of the Centennial Trail off of Northwest Boulevard would be faced with another condition placed on it by Union Pacific Railroad. UP denied an at-grade crossing of the railroad track. The railroad tracks were between Northwest Boulevard and the Spokane River. The trail had to cross the train tracks to be on the west side of the corridor and nearer to the river. Trail users would have to go on a bridge or through a tunnel to get to the rails with trails location. Estimates on either of these crossings would cost an additional $250,000.00 to $400,000.00.

Headquarters for Union Pacific Railroad was located in Kansas. Long distance communication proved ineffective in resolving this latest issue. The railroad insisted that an at-grade crossing would not be allowed regardless of the signage that the trail organizers offered to install. Building a tunnel or a bridge that may not be used in a few short years if the rumors of railroad track abandonment were true, did not make financial sense.

The trail was held up from making this connection for the better part of another year.

In February of 2002 the City of Coeur d'Alene hired a new attorney, Mike Gridley. Mike was an avid bicyclist and had recently completed a bicycle ride from coast to coast. He also shared the vision of expanded pedestrian and bicycle routes throughout the community. The company, Mike had worked for, offered early buy-outs, or early retirements, to long term employees. He took them up on the offer even though he was too young to consider retirement. The company he had worked for was Union Pacific Railroad.

A few months after settling into his new job, Mike offered to see what he could do to mitigate the nearly one-year stalemate on the trail and rail crossing. By the latter part of the summer of 2002 the issue had been resolved. Neither a bridge, nor a tunnel, would be necessary. The trail would have the appropriate signage warning users of the railroad crossing.

The city applied for, and was awarded, a Transportation Equity Act for the 21st Century grant (TEA-21), also known as the Transportation Enhancement Act, to relocate the trail onto this corridor near the Spokane River. Awarding of the grant, preparing trail construction documents, bidding and contracting placed this section of trail development in 2003. This new section of trail was opened in 2004.

By 2006 the Union Pacific railroad tracks across the BLM property and through the Riverstone subdivision were removed and the line was abandoned. The City of Coeur d'Alene, Ignite CDA and the North Idaho Centennial Trail Foundation acquired the abandoned railroad property west of Riverstone. This corridor extended five miles west and north toward the Rathdrum Prairie. A 15-foot-wide paved pedestrian/bicycle trail was built on the abandoned railroad corridor that connects to the Centennial Trail. Mike Gridley was instrumental in the land acquisition and development of this trail extension which is known as the Prairie Trail.

Mullan Avenue in Coeur d'Alene was yet another problem area for the trail committee, the only Class III trail along the 23-mile route. The trail travels along Mullan Avenue from 8th Street to 23rd Street, or what is now called Coeur d'Alene Lake Drive. Residents on Mullan Avenue access their garages from an alley way. Parking on the street was where visitors would park as well as the home owners. The trail developers recommended that one side of Mullan become a no-parking zone and that a Class II trail be established on the south side of the street. The residents and the City Council were not comfortable with that proposal and allowed parking to remain on both sides of the street. This created a shared use of the roadway with vehicles, pedestrians and bicyclists.

Throughout most of the 1990's, this section of the trail was discussed frequently. There were no sidewalks on either side of Mullan Avenue and pedestrians had to use the road to travel along the trail route.

In the spring of 2000, the city council authorized 'no-parking' signs on the south side of Mullan Avenue as a pilot program. This action made for a safer corridor and eliminated the only Class III section of the Centennial Trail. Recommendations were later made to prohibit parking on both sides of Mullan Avenue but that was denied.

In 2011-2012 the State of Idaho agreed to construct an on-ramp/off-ramp at mile one on Interstate 90. This agreement was in conjunction with Cabela's building a store on the Idaho side of the Washington/Idaho border. The construction of the new interchange interrupted the trail for over a year. The Idaho Transportation Department managed the project and the end result was very favorable for the trail

In 2016 the City of Coeur d'Alene entertained the idea of liquidating part of the Centennial Trail corridor west of Beebe Boulevard in the Riverstone subdivision. The purpose was to allow for housing in this corridor potentially generating funds from the sale of the land. The trail foundation informed the city council that this action would have a negative impact on trail users and the Riverstone community. The trail would be reduced from 15 feet in width to 9 feet in width and relocated away from Riverstone Park. The proximate principle was also used to identify that a trail greenbelt in this corridor would increase property values. The property value increase would result in a return of revenue that would prove to be greater, in the long run, than the sale of the land. The council withdrew this idea of selling the land and entered into an agreement with the trail foundation that would allow for a trail greenbelt through this area. The greenbelt may ultimately traverse along, or near, the riverfront from Beebe Boulevard in Riverstone for one mile west to Huetter Road.

An issue, or problem, will inevitably pop-up along the 23-mile trail route that will impact the experience for the trail user. The trail foundation and governing entities along the trail strive to minimize trail disruptions ensuring a safe, enjoyable use of the North Idaho Centennial Trail.

Chapter 17
Rails to Trails

    Back in the 1920's, the railroads had reached their peak with over 275,000 miles of rail tracks throughout the country. Between 1935 and 1975, nearly 40,000 miles of those rail tracks were abandoned. Congress passed the Staggers Rail Act in 1980, making it easier for railroads to abandon unused corridors. This triggered a greater amount of rail abandonment than was anticipated. Over the course of the next 15 years, nearly 65,000 additional miles of railroad lines would be abandoned.[11] "Railbanking" was the term used and it allowed for other types of transportation to occur on the abandoned railroad corridors without forfeiting the future use of the corridor for railroads or other necessary transportation. Thus, came the pedestrian and bicycle trails which led to the introduction of the Rail to Trail Conservancy (RTC). The RTC was officially opened in 1986. In their first year, they helped secure 250 miles of railroad property for trails. Today over 25,000 miles of railroad corridors have become recreational trails throughout the country.

    The North Idaho Centennial Trail uses several sections of abandoned railroad along its 23-mile path. Starting at the state line, there are five acres of railroad property on both sides of the old historic bridge that crosses the Spokane River. About one mile east of there, the Centennial Trail travels along another three miles of abandoned railroad right of way. The City of Post Falls recently added another section to the trail, extending

---

[11] Rails to Trails Conservancy 2011 History of Railroads

from Spokane Street to Greensferry Road, about three more miles of old railroad property.

In Coeur d'Alene, the railroad did not own all the land directly under their tracks. They had a long term, renewable lease that would remain in effect until they had no more clients along the railroad route. The majority of those clients were lumber mills.

Starting in 1989, lumber mills began to close down their operations along the Spokane River and banks of Lake Coeur d'Alene as demand for lumber declined. The first one to close was the Rutledge/Potlatch mill on the east side of the city. The last one to close was near North Idaho College in 2008. This mill was owned and operated by Stimson Lumber Company, formerly DeArmond Mill. Stimson bought Idaho Forest Industries and DeArmond just five years earlier. The mill produced 2 X 4 and 2 X 6 studs.

Once the last mill was closed, the railroads began the process of abandoning those corridors. Since the railroads did not own the land under the tracks, the land reverted back to the original owner, which was the United States Government. Nearly one mile of the abandoned lines became the property of the Bureau of Land Management (BLM). The BLM gave permission to install the trail on the railroad right of way in Coeur d'Alene.

Two well-known trails in North Idaho were established as a direct result of the Rails to Trails Conservancy. The Hiawatha Trail runs 13 miles, connecting Idaho to Montana. It is managed by the U.S. Forrest Service and offers spectacular views, trestles and tunnels. The Taft Tunnel on this trail (named after President William H. Taft) is 1.7 miles long. This is an unpaved trail with a 2% grade from Idaho to Montana. The Hiawatha Trail opened in 1998 after a bit of a struggle with the timber industry. This particular rail corridor was being acquired by the timber industry to log and move equipment in the back country. The U.S. Forest Service objected to this sale and eventually secured the rail corridor.

The Trail of the Coeur d'Alene's is a 72-mile paved trail that travels from the town of Mullan in the Silver Valley, to the City of Plummer in the Coeur d'Alene Indian Reservation. The Coeur d'Alene Tribe sued Union Pacific Railroad for contaminants along the trail corridor in 1999. The railroad eventually had to clean up the corridor and compensated the tribe by building the trail. The section of the trail on tribal land is managed by the Coeur d'Alene Tribe. The section of the Trail of the Coeur d'Alene's that is outside of the reservation is managed by the State of Idaho Parks and Recreation Department. The Trail of the Coeur d'Alene's officially opened to the public in 2004.

This 72-mile trail also became targeted to become part of a proposed National Trail System, the Great American Rail Trail. The Rails to Trails Conservancy proposed to connect a trail system from Seattle, Washington to the Washington D.C. area. The length of this national trail system is estimated to be 3,700 miles. A great portion of this proposed trail is already in place, with some missing sections scattered across the country. The efforts of the RTC included reacquiring those missing sections of railroad property and ultimately have a coast-to-coast trail system.

As of today, 2019-2020, approximately ten miles of property are required to connect the Trail of the Coeur d'Alene's with the Palouse to the Cascades Trail in Washington (formerly the John Wayne Trail). Bit by bit it will come together, and that will be one great legacy for many generations.

The RTC was also instrumental in lobbying congress for the introduction of the TEA-21 (Transportation Enhancement Act) and ISTEA (Interstate Transportation Enhancement Act) funding grants. These grants are allocated through the federal government and administered by individual state transportation departments. Coeur d'Alene received two of these grants. The first one was for the Centennial Trail parking lot at Northwest Boulevard and Seltice Way. The grant included beautification of the I-90 Interchange in that same area.

The second grant allowed for the development of the Centennial Trail on the BLM site that led from the east side of the Riverstone development to North Idaho College. This latter development and grant opportunity proved to be very timely, as the City of Coeur d'Alene had recently rebuilt Northwest Boulevard from the I-90 Interchange into town. The original Centennial Trail route traveled on Northwest Boulevard, but it was not included in the rebuilt Northwest Boulevard plan. There was some temporary trail interruption but it quickly resolved for the better, through cooperation from the BLM, transportation grants, and the City of Coeur d'Alene.

Chapter 18
Naming A Premier Idaho Trail

The North Idaho Centennial Trail was initially referred to as 'the trail,' a non-descript name that could have applied to any trail project, anywhere in America. This project, the concept of a bi-state trail, was introduced to the Kootenai County Centennial Committee in 1987.

The Governor of Idaho, Phil Batt, requested that each of the 44 counties in Idaho establish a centennial committee to prepare for the state's 100th birthday in 1990. The trail project was endorsed by the committee and was later proposed as the 'Centennial Trail,' a lasting legacy to the citizenry in honor of the state's centennial. However, the Idaho Department of Parks and Recreation had already named a trail project that they were proposing as the Centennial Trail. Their project charted a course for people to hike from the Idaho/Utah border to the Idaho/Canadian border. The State Parks trail had already been endorsed by the state centennial commission, so the trail planners in Kootenai County renamed their project. Two words were added to the name; 'North Idaho'. The project became known as the North Idaho Centennial Trail.

Spokane was actively charting and planning their state's adjoining trail route. They were in negotiations with the Inland Empire Paper Company to trade land with Spokane County. Fortunately, they were able to agree to a land trade that would provide Spokane County with river frontage, through the Spokane Valley and into the city. When the land trade was completed, they named their trail system the Spokane River Centennial Trail. Spokane would construct a trail 39 miles in length and Idaho would connect to that with an additional 23 miles of trail, creating a consecutive 62-mile trail system.

The Spokane trail supporters had also designed a logo for their trail. The logo represented trees, the river, and a trail. The goal of both state trail supporters was to have the trails connect, making this trail the largest trail system in the area. Supporters from both states thought it would be a good idea for trail users, traversing from state to state, to have continuity in signage. The Idaho Trail Committee requested permission from the Spokane Trail Committee, to use the same logo design through both states, which was granted. The color scheme was changed on the North Idaho Centennial Trail. Trail users from Spokane to Coeur d'Alene can readily identify that they are on the Centennial Trail by these visible logo signs.

Chapter 19
Millennium Legacy Trail

The North Idaho Centennial Trail was recognized as a Millennium Legacy Trail ten years after the initial ground-breaking. Only one trail in each of the 50 states would receive this recognition. In 1998-99, the White House began preparation for the upcoming Millennium for the year 2000.

One of the many things being promoted at that time to celebrate this event, was to recognize the trail systems across the country. The White House Millennium Council, the U.S. Department of Transportation, and the Rails to Trails Conservancy became partners to implement this program. The White House stated that the Millennium Trails' initiative was to recognize, promote, and support trails that preserve open space, interpret history and culture, and embrace recreation and tourism. Every state was invited to nominate trails within their respective states. The governor of each state picked one trail system to be submitted to the White House for Millennium Trail Status recognition.

Every community in our state was invited to submit a recommendation to the Governor's office for consideration of this national honor. Dave Fair, the Post Falls Parks and Recreation Director, suggested that the North Idaho Centennial Trail be submitted for consideration. Phil Batt, the Governor in 1999, submitted the North Idaho Centennial Trail as the trail project to represent Idaho. The Boise Greenbelt was also a candidate, along with other submissions. It is important to note that the North Idaho Centennial Trail was the longest pedestrian/bicycle trail system in the state, at that time, connecting several communities and two states.

On November 17, 1999, the State of Idaho received a letter from the secretary of the U.S. Department of Transportation, stating that the North Idaho Centennial Trail had been designated as one of the fifty Millennium Legacy Trails. The secretary went on to say, "*The Millennium Legacy Trail status symbolizes the spirit of our efforts to connect our nation's culture, heritage and communities. The Millennium Legacy Trails will provide a route for children to walk to school, for commuters to ride to work and for travelers of all ages and abilities to see and feel a connection to America's past. I can think of no finer legacy than to leave to our children and our children's children this network of historic trails.*"

The North Idaho Centennial Trail is highly used, greatly appreciated, and now you know it is also recognized on a national level as a Millennium Legacy Trail.

Another interesting note about the North Idaho Centennial Trail is that it can be said that three United States Presidents have their fingerprints on this great trail.

- 1988: President Ronald Regan signed the federal budget that allowed for partial funding for the North Idaho Centennial Trail and the Spokane River Centennial Trail.
- 1990: President George Bush was invited by Speaker of the House Tom Foley to come to Spokane and help us dedicate the centennial trails. President Bush was in route to Seattle and accepted the offer to help dedicate the trail.
- 2000: President Clinton's white house administration had implemented a Millennium Trail Legacy

recognizing the upcoming millennium. The North Idaho Centennial Trail received the honor.

Chapter 20
North Idaho Centennial Trail Foundation

The North Idaho Centennial Trail Foundation began as the Centennial Trail oversight committee in 1989. As the Coeur d'Alene Parks Director, I pitched the idea of creating this committee to assist the three owner agencies with the long-term care of the trail. Even though there was a high degree of controversy surrounding the trail project, including the freezing of development funds, I remained optimistic the trail would be completed. I also recognized that, at some point in the future, capital improvement funds would be needed to preserve the Centennial Trail. With this in mind, I requested that each of the three owner entities allocate an equal, agreed upon dollar amount annually, that would go directly to the trail budget account. In addition, the trail committee would raise funds designated to the long-term care account. The funds would be allowed to accrue and draw interest. All three entities implemented this plan in fiscal year 1990-91, and have continued to contribute to the long-term care fund.

Also, in 1989, as the state's centennial committees were winding down, the North Idaho Centennial Trail Chairman, Bob Nelson, suggested that the committee become a foundation and seek 501(c)3 tax status from the Internal Revenue Service (IRS), making it a recognized non-profit organization. The Centennial Trail was promoted as a lasting legacy to the community, and the project was adopted by the county centennial committee. However, unlike most of the centennial celebration ideas, the trail would live on, and on, and could use the 501(c)3 status for fund raising purposes. Nelson said he would file the paperwork with the IRS seeking the non-profit possibility. In late 1989, the IRS approved the request for the committee to become the North Idaho Centennial Trail Foundation.

The North Idaho Centennial Trail Foundation (NICTF) is comprised of 18 board members who meet monthly. The NICTF has several sub-committees that may meet more often and have dozens more volunteers involved, depending on the project or status of upcoming fundraising events. In addition to the NICTF, a Joint Powers Board (JPB) was established to work closely with the foundation on the long-term care and capital improvements for the trail.

The JPB is comprised of an elected official, such as a county commissioner or city council member, from each of the three entities. They meet semi-annually with the NICTF to review the budget and discuss long-term capital improvements, which are projected out for 5 years. A maintenance committee for the trail meets quarterly with staff representatives from each of the entities and board members from the NICTF. This group assures continuity along the 23-mile trail with regard to trail surface, signage, weed control, and everything else that promotes enjoyable use of the Centennial Trail.

The NICTF Board of Directors is comprised of individuals having a variety of business and community backgrounds, and more importantly, are dedicated users of the trail. They contribute valuable information, and insight, based on personal experience. To that end, the NICTF Board is probably the best, 'free,' service the community has available for input on design, development, and long-term care of a pedestrian and bicycle trail.

The North Idaho Centennial Trail Foundation Board of Directors is currently looking into lighting the old historic railroad bridge at the state line, more commonly known today as the North Idaho Centennial Trail Bridge. The foundation board has also drawn-up plans to create a greenbelt along the Centennial Trail in Riverstone. This plan also identifies the concept of capturing the railroad history that traversed through the community connecting our historical towns. The NICTF Board recently completed an economic impact study on how the trail brings new money into the community, and enhances the value of property along the trail corridor.

More information about the North Idaho Centennial Trail and the North Idaho Centennial Trail Foundation can be found on their website at www.nictf.org.
If you are interested in becoming a board member, or a volunteer, on any of the NICTF committees, please contact them through the web site.

Chapter 21
23 STORIES

Told by Individuals That Have Enjoyed and Experienced the Centennial Trail

Ever since the North Idaho Centennial Trail had been completed, it is enjoyed by hundreds of thousands of walkers, runners and bicyclists every year. Stories are told by individuals of their adventures and appreciation of this magnificent trail system. One day Tabitha Kraack mentioned that we, the NICTF Board, should gather these stories in writing. She added that we should collect 23 stories, one for each mile of the trail and publish the stories in our newsletter. The idea gained traction, and it was decided that we would reach out to the community, seek the individual stories and add them to the trail book. The COVID Pandemic prevented the foundation board from doing a community wide 30-year celebration, and a second edition to the book would be a nice amenity for the belated 30-year celebration.

David Groth, North Idaho Centennial Trail Board member liked the idea, and volunteered to collect these heartwarming stories for the second edition to the North Idaho Centennial Trail – The Trail That Almost Wasn't.

A special thanks to the individuals that took the time to share their stories with all of us.

Training on the Centennial Trail
by Alan Wolfe

    An Ironman race is daunting. A 2.4-mile swim, a 112-mile bike ride, and a full 26.2-mile marathon, all in the same day. Daunting.... but not as hard as you think. What could be harder?
The training.
The race itself is one day. The training is 140 days, and that doesn't count getting in shape to start the actual Ironman training program.
    In the case of Ironman Coeur d'Alene, that training started in February in North Idaho. Those five months include some of the nastiest weather that you will see throughout the year. Some of the training can be done inside but after a few weeks staring at a wall on your cycling trainer, you need to get outside, or you will go bonkers.
    I am extremely fortunate to live a half-mile from the Centennial Trail, which was a godsend to me and my training. What many people don't know is the maintenance that is performed throughout the winter on the trail. After slipping, and sliding, to get to the trail, it was so nice to have miles, and miles, of clean, smooth asphalt to focus on training, and not falling on my...
    Since my training program called for 2500+ miles of cycling, and 500+ miles of running, I needed to have this safe environment in which to work. Anyone who has done much cycling on the road will tell you, not all motorists "share the road", or are the least bit interested in moving over to give you, and your bike, plenty of room to maneuver.
    Once again, the Centennial Trail provided a super safe place to train, and focus, on getting the job done

rather than stress about staying alive. It is also a beautiful place to help pass the many hours you need to get the job done. I would oftentimes come home with my daily "bunny count" as I would record the number of baby bunnies I would see along my way. It was a lot more fun than just simply counting miles.

To those in charge, and those who support the Centennial Trail, ... Thank You ... for providing me, and countless others, with such a wonderful place to train.

Central To My Life
by Amy Wearne

    The Centennial Trail has been a staple go-to for myself, my family, and my fitness community for as long as I can remember.
    Personally, I use the trail for running while I train for local endurance races, or destination races. My family has also been taking full advantage of the trail for riding bikes. I have a 9-year-old, and a 7-year-old, so the trail has offered us a way to get from one part of town to another on bikes, as well as a way to spend time together while I'm training! Whether it's meeting a girlfriend early in the morning for a beautiful walk, and great conversation, or plugging in my headphones to attack a hard training session, it provides the perfect backdrop to capture the beautiful place in which we live.
    I have led a 'running club' for several years, and one of our most common places to meet is on Coeur d'Alene Lake Drive. We have done every type of workout on that trail, and there was even a time that I had to hop in a car, and drive back to get people, because I had a 'miss' on my programming, and people were way too far out to make it back to work on time!
    I also own AIM Nutrition Coaching, and at the beginning of the year, we rallied members to sign up for the CDA Half Marathon. Due to COVID-19, our race was canceled but our members were still determined to achieve a goal they had set, so we continued to prepare as a community for #aimrunsahalfmarathon, which took place the day before we would have run the CDA Half! Our members took full advantage of the Centennial Trail during the last three months of their training, and accomplished a goal many of them never thought was

possible, most of them never having run a half marathon before!

I grew up in Coeur d'Alene, and began using the trail as a child. When I think about my adult life, the overwhelming memories come from the two full Coeur d'Alene Ironman races, which were completed on a good chunk of the Centennial Trail! The years I spent training on the trails, from Tuesday night 60-mile rides, where we would take turns 'pulling' out to Higgens Point to turning around and doing a 'brick workout,' where we then fought up Bennett Bay hill by foot...Ironman memories are ingrained in my heart.

As an eight-year-old, my dad, brother, and I set out to ride our bikes from Hayden, Idaho to Lake Roosevelt. I remember getting a flat tire at the start of the Centennial Trail...we had hardly crossed town to start our adventure and we already had our first flat! We used the Centennial Trail all the way to Riverstone Park in Spokane, before heading onto Highway 2 for the remainder of our adventure.

I can even remember using the portion of the trail out to Higgens Point on Ironman race day as a way to track my race nutrition. Making sure that by the time I was on my way back in from Higgens, I had consumed Cliff Bar number one, and drank half of water bottle number one. I can even remember my dad driving alongside me as I ran up Bennett Bay, holding a sign, yelling for me to "stick with it!" Or in my second Ironman, checking on a friend I was about to pass as he was forced to walk due to cramps. Needless to say, I have very distinct, pride-filled memories on that trail because two of the biggest athletic accomplishments I've ever had involved me grinding through miles, and miles, on the Centennial Trail.

I've ridden the entire 23-miles of the trail many times. When I was training, and doing "century rides" (100-mile rides), there was a lot of ground to cover. Another common ride was the well-known Rocket Ride in the Ironman community. Starting in Idaho, we would ride the Centennial Trail into Eastern Washington to the Rocket Bakery Café, enjoy their sweet baked goods, and ride back into Idaho, and home. That was a staple in our training!

The trail has given me the freedom, and opportunity, to train for athletic events that most people don't dream of doing. The Centennial Trail has also offered me a continued sense of community, and happiness, as I use it with my family, and within my professional life.

THE TRAIL THAT ALMOST WASN'T

Volunteer Clean-Up
by Bob Forsythe

I grew up in Coeur d'Alene after moving here from Eastern Montana with my family, and have lived here ever since, except for 20 years while I served in the Navy, and got to see areas throughout Asia, and the Eastern African coast. I saw totally filthy, and littered countries, as well as Singapore, one of the world's cleanest cities.

Upon retiring from the Navy, I returned to college at North Idaho College. where I obtained a degree in Law Enforcement. I then received a job with the Kootenai County Sheriff's Office as a Detention Deputy. I worked there for 15 years, achieving the rank of sergeant.

In this capacity, I worked three years as the Work Release Supervisor, and was responsible for the Sheriff's Community Labor Program. One of the programs I managed was the roadside litter pick-up. I always felt a sense of pride, and accomplishment, on how this program benefited our community.

After retiring from the sheriff's office, I started to appreciate, and enjoy, the Centennial Trail in earnest. I initially started walking the trail from Tony's Restaurant parking area to Steamer Crossing. I noticed trash laying along the trail, and roadway, day after day for the first week.

At the end of the first week, I observed three syringes discarded in the grass at Steamer Crossing Rest Area. I told myself, "Enough is enough!" Realizing this area was utilized by families, and pet owners, I went out and bought my first gripper, and a box of 13-gallon kitchen trash bags. I then decided to do my part: Titus 2:7 *"And you yourself must be an example to them by doing good works of every kind. Let everything you do reflect the integrity and seriousness of your teaching."*

In the next three-plus years, I continued doing these walks. I have worn out six grippers, and emptied three boxes of trash bags! I figured I might as well do something positive for my community, and home. I unofficially adopted a stretch of the Centennial Trail from the Fernan Lake drainage pond (city limits) to the trails of Higgens Point, where I can be located most mornings.

I have expanded my clean up efforts to occasionally clean other areas, such as Post Falls' Treaty Rock Park, Q'emilin Park, the Falls Park, Corbin Park, and Fernan Lake Natural Area. All of these areas are close to the Centennial Trail. My efforts assist our community parks, the Eastside Highway District, the citizens of Kootenai County, and those who visit our area for events such as the Coeur d'Alene marathon, Ironman, and eagle watching. 1 Peter 4:10 *"As each has received a gift, use it to serve one another."*

As previously stated, I initially started to walk the trail for personal health reasons, then progressed to community service, and awareness. I have met many people on the trail who asked me why I pick up the trash others leave behind. My answer is simple, "I do it for you, so you can enjoy the spectacular views, and because this is my home, and I am proud of its beauty!"

THE TRAIL THAT ALMOST WASN'T

Wrong Restroom
by Chris Guggemos
written by David Groth

"One Saturday a group of Panhandle Kiwanis members invited me to bicycle from Coeur d'Alene to Riverfront Park in Spokane. Maybe it was even a little past that?" said Chris Guggemos.

It was a beautiful day, with much of the ride on the Centennial Trail. We traveled west out of Coeur d'Alene along I-90, through Post Falls, and next to the Spokane River. It was by far the longest bicycle ride Chris had ever done, and when he arrived at Riverfront Park he thought, "And now I have to ride back?!"

After a bit of rest, the group cruised east toward Coeur d'Alene for at least ten miles before stopping at a rest area near Mirabeau Park in the Spokane Valley. Chris used the restroom and when he came out, he noticed his friends seemed somewhat amused, and saw them pointing at the sign on the door: "Ladies". Chris was extremely tired, too tired to notice any signs.

He survived that embarrassment, and forced himself to ride on for another ten miles until they arrived at the Pleasant View intersection in Post Falls. "I was on fumes," Chris said, and he thought seriously about sticking out his thumb on I-90, and hitching a ride back to Coeur d'Alene. But he didn't.

Chris made it home after about 80 miles of cycling, "Having never been more exhausted!" This was the start of his interest in cycling, and it led to a better bicycle, a used Trek that he got from Doug Eastwood.

Months later, Chris decided to ride to the state line, near the Pleasant View intersection. He cruised west on The Centennial Trail and was feeling great, amazed at how effortless it seemed. And then he turned toward home, and the intense head wind taught him quickly why the ride west had been so easy.

"I wasn't riding to get exercise. I just didn't have anything to do," said Chris. So, without any hesitation, he detoured toward I-90, stuck out his thumb, and hopped in a pickup truck that brought him all the way back to his home in Coeur d'Alene.

Chris smiled and added, "I'm not sure I've ever told Doug this story."

THE TRAIL THAT ALMOST WASN'T

The Walking Guy
by Darrell Dlouhy

There was a period of time in my life when I'd walk the trail every day. I did this for nearly five years. I've lost track. I'd walk from the first parking area just beyond the beautiful condos east of CDA. I'd continue on to the top of the hill just beyond Tony's restaurant. The total walk: about 5 miles.

I'd walk no matter what the weather. I'd walk in the summer heat, and even on the most bitter cold days of winter. I went for a walk every day. I've only recently come to find out I was dubbed "the walking guy" by those that lived out in that area. I remember, occasionally, in the heat of summer, having to intrude on a "private "dock and jump in the lake to cool down. In contrast, I remember on the blusteriest, and wickedly days of winter, leaning into the bitingly cold winds as I headed back to my car, cursing under my breath as if my disdain could tame winter's fury.

Even now, many years later, I fondly remember these daily walks and each familiar turn, or tree, or dock, or house on the hillside as my companion. That Centennial Trail is our treasure. That portion of our trail had the power to draw me day after day, year after year, to take in its beauty.

Wouldn't It Be Great . . .
by David Groth

In 1983 I lived on Sunnyside Road, east of Coeur d'Alene. Most days I rode my bicycle down the half mile hill and then hugged Lake Coeur d'Alene for two more miles to town, on what was then Interstate 90.

It was a beautiful ride, despite cars, and trucks, whizzing by at 65 mile per hour. I enjoyed seeing the different moods of the lake, and often the symmetric line of deciduous trees, rooted between the south shoulder of the interstate, and the lake. The trees would sway in the wind. Every day I thought, "What an incredible location this would be for a bike trail?!"

And then it happened. In 1987, construction was completed on the 240-foot Veterans Memorial Centennial Bridge. The bridge spanned the water overlooking Lake Coeur d'Alene's Bennett Bay, which was the last link in rerouting Interstate 90 to a location above the lake, rather than hugging the shore. With that historical event, the former location of Interstate 90 was transformed to quiet Coeur d'Alene Lake Drive, and also referred to as the Lake Coeur d'Alene Scenic Byway.

During the construction of the bridge and new roadway, I heard rumblings of my dream for a trail along the north shore of Lake Coeur d'Alene, and then confirmation that it was in process. In 1990 I took my first bike ride on the North Idaho Centennial Trail from Post Falls to the Idaho/Washington state line. My dream was indeed being fulfilled. In 1995, the trail along the east shore of the lake had been completed, and the Centennial Trail, all 23 miles, was connected from Coeur d'Alene (Higgins Point) to Spokane, Washington.

THE TRAIL THAT ALMOST WASN'T

Since then, I've cycled from Coeur d'Alene to Higgins Point hundreds of times, have hiked the same 5 1/2 mile stretch many times. I competed in two Ironman races on the eastern part of the Centennial Trail. I have cross country skied on this same section, shared conversations with friends while sitting on benches along the trail, and have used the Centennial Trail to access swimming spots along the lake. I ride the trail to get to The Kroc Center and occasionally start there and walk or cycle the western part of the Centennial Trail, sometimes connecting with The Prairie Trail.

In 2016 I retired as a teacher in Coeur d'Alene. While discussing with a college friend my plans to retire, he commented, "If there's something physical that you want to do, NOW is probably the time."

With that nudge, I focused on a long-time dream of taking a significant cycling trip, and decided to ride the west coast, from Coeur d'Alene to San Diego. After months of enjoyably solidifying plans, in September of 2016, six friends escorted me out of Coeur d'Alene on the Centennial Trail. After lunch at the Rocket Bakery in Spokane, my friends cycled back to Coeur d'Alene, and I continued west on The Centennial Trail. Once again, the trail was a kickoff to fulfilling a dream.

So Many Uses . . .
by Deb

I first started walking the Centennial Trail when I moved from Cougar Gulch to the downtown Coeur d'Alene area. That was in 1989, and by late 1991, I was pushing a stroller, pulling my toddler on a sled and cruising around with him on the back of my bicycle. The "new library" was not yet built and the trail looked very different, but it was always wonderful, and convenient, to walk out my door, and be on a safe, and beautiful trail through town, and by the lake.

As our son grew up, we biked, roller-skated, and skateboarded along the trail in both directions. There were even winters when I would put on my cross-country skis, and ski out my door, down the trail, through the City Park and along the lake! Every season has its own challenges, and beauty, from icy patches, and crowds of outdoor enthusiasts to the colors, and beauty of the mountains, trees and water. I have always felt so lucky, and blessed, to live in Coeur d'Alene, and have access to so much. It never gets old!

A Thirty-Year Journey
by Denise Lundy

A Thirty-year journey of pedaling, and playing, on the North Idaho Centennial Trail.

In the early 1990s, I relocated from Bellevue, Washington, to downtown Coeur d'Alene. I spent my youth capitalizing on the Sammamish River, and Burke Gilman Trail network, around Lake Sammamish, and Lake Washington. I loved cycling along the Sammamish Slough through Marymoor Park and around Lake Washington into the city. Alas, I found Washington's west side, and the trails I cherished had become too crowded for my taste.

When I discovered North Idaho, I instantly fell in love with the region for its stunning landscape, friendly residents, and pristine lakes. Fleeing a more populous area, I was delighted by the uncrowded trailheads in North Idaho. Phase I of the 23-mile Centennial Trail was under construction. I knew this trail system would be a gem to the community, and it played a big part in my relocation to the Lake City.

As a new resident, I rollerbladed (no judgment, it was the early 1990s) up and down the lake's shore on the North Idaho Centennial Trail's smooth new asphalt. Over the years, I became familiar with and explored this trail from end to end. By 1995, when the 23-mile trail was completed, I would run, or cycle, through Sanders Beach to Higgens Point after work, and explored the portions of the trail along the Spokane River on the weekends. Longer rides extended into the Washington portion of the Centennial Trail through the city of Spokane, and into Riverside State Park.

My second decade as a trail user was quite different from the first. We have all heard countless stories of parents taking their infant for a car ride to soothe, or put their baby to sleep. My daughter was born a child that abhorred the automobile. Any car trip involved relentless, ear-piercing screams that sent me into tears! As a result, I parked my car for the better part of two years and fell back on my old friend, the North Idaho Centennial Trail. I pulled my infant daughter in the Burley bike trailer, and carried her for walks in the backpack all along the Centennial Trail, mom, and baby, both contented.

It was not long before my daughter learned to walk, and walk we did around Tubbs Hill, and along the Lake on the Centennial trail every day. A few years later, it was on the Centennial Trail that I taught my daughter to ride a bike along Coeur d'Alene Lake Drive. It was a picture-perfect setting to capture both her proud grin of success, and the sparkling lake in the background.

We had many visitors during those years, and whether welcoming a guest, client, or relative to Coeur d'Alene always included a stroll, or bike ride on the Centennial Trail. I enjoyed being a tourist in my own backyard, and watching people take in the splendor of this trail for the first time, perhaps on a walk from the Coeur d'Alene Resort past the City Beach, and around the historic Fort Grounds neighborhood.

By the end of this decade, my daughter and I were running organized fun runs together on the trail.

My third decade as a Centennial Trail user was markedly different from the prior twenty years. Compelled to give back to the trail I loved, I served on the North Idaho Centennial Trail Foundation board for many years. Still, I received more from this trail than I was ever able to repay. I formed many long-lasting friendships with other trail supporters, and board members. Getting to know these forward-thinking pioneers determined to bring this trail to fruition was humbling, and deeply gratifying.

I enjoyed helping to organize, and participating, in the NICTF's fundraisers, and events. Riding the Coeur d'Fondo, and sipping pints at Ales for the Trail, I learned first-hand that even in divisive, or tumultuous times, the trail brings people together mile by mile, and smile by smile.

As empty-nesters my husband, and I, frequently cycle to Higgens Point, and walk our Golden Doodle on the trail. While I have long since retired my rollerblades, I now use my roller skis on the trail in the fall to prepare for the winter's Nordic ski season.

When my father comes to visit, we cycle together on the trail, only now I struggle to keep up with him when he engages the assist on his shiny new e-bike up the Bennet Bay Hill!

The trail has been a multi-generational playground for my family. I am eternally grateful for the memories of keeping active, parenting, and forming lasting friendships along the North Idaho Centennial Trail. Cheers!

Starting at Age Six
by Derek Garcia

My memories of growing up in Coeur d' Alene wouldn't be complete without the adventures, training, and events that have taken place on the North Idaho Centennial Trail.

When I was six years old, I did a five-hour, 23-mile bike ride with my father that included stops along Lake Coeur d' Alene, and the Spokane River. My dad brought our lunch, and we rode the entire North Idaho portion to the Washington/ Idaho state line, where some friends picked us up. I remember being exhausted, and sunburnt, and I also felt so accomplished to have ridden such a long way at age six. In comparison to this earlier summer ride, I recall the next fall, and how easy it was to ride my bike three miles to school.

By the time I was in college I had gotten a bit out of shape, which started the transition from my high school athletic days to becoming a professional triathlete. During the summer after my first year of college, I completed a six-mile bike ride along the Higgens Point section of the Centennial Trail. This was done on a mountain bike with partially flat tires, which further emphasized how out of shape I had become. But who knew that within 15 years I would bike nearly 1,000 miles, just on that portion of the trail!

Finishing my first Coeur d'Alene Olympic Distance Triathlon after endless hours of biking, and running, completing my first Ironman, and ultimately becoming one of the top triathletes in the world, started with riding, and running, along The Centennial Trail. Whether it was serious training, or the best way to kick off the year at the Hangover Handicap Five-Mile Run, the Centennial Trail has been central to my life in Northern Idaho. My three boys now hear those stories, and they are excited to ride the trail with me this coming summer. Maybe we can even hit all 23 miles.

How It All Began!
by Evalyn Adams

In 1986, when Governor Cecil Andrus, and State Centennial Chairman, Harry Magnuson, asked Counties in Idaho to help oversee State Centennial activities, I volunteered to lead the effort for Kootenai County. I was the only Commissioner at that time who had been born in Idaho, and was eager to assist with this special one-hundred-year celebration. Idaho received its statehood in 1890. The governor had put in motion, a few years ahead of our states' centennial, plans for Idaho to celebrate in a big way in 1990. I was also the County Commissioner who had volunteered to take the lead on parks and waterways facilities in the County.

After an earlier '86 fall meeting in Spokane with people interested in exploring the concept of a two state Centennial Trail, a meeting was held back in Coeur d'Alene. Some of those attending included City Councilman Bob McDonald, and CDA Parks Director Doug Eastwood. Post Falls was represented by City Councilwoman Karen Streeter.

I was excited about Centennial opportunities, and attended both meetings, and felt very positive about working on the two state Trail. I had lived in Boise, Idaho and Eugene, Oregon where both cities had developed wonderful trail systems along the water. My family had used these recreational opportunities and I felt northern Idaho deserved to have a great trail, and it would be an outstanding Centennial project. Even though Washington's Centennial was in 1989, the year before Idaho's, people from both states felt it should be a joint venture.

With support from Kootenai County and the cities of Coeur d'Alene, and Post Falls, a trail committee was formed, and plans were formulated about the route, and funding possibilities. The two cities jointly financed a trail master plan. John Muller of Architects West/Landmark was the lead person on the project. After attending many of the meetings, I decided to concentrate on trail funding efforts.

In 1987 I made plans to attend a national meeting for County Commissioners in Washington D.C., and met with Spokane lady Commissioner Pat Mummy, who was supportive of the Centennial Trail effort. Mummy arranged a meeting with Tom Foley, who was Speaker of the House, and she and I met with Foley in his office. He sounded very supportive, and I met separately with Idaho's Senators Jim McClure and Steve Symms to acquaint them with this exciting opportunity. I also stopped by Congressman Larry Craig's office to gain his support.

Before being elected County Commissioner in 1985, I had served eight years as executive officer of the North Idaho Building Contractors Association (NIBCA). In that position, I attended meetings of the National Association of Home Builders in Washington D.C. and had become acquainted with Idaho's Congressional delegation. I always tried to connect with some of their staff during visits because they quite often would help when I had questions. Both Senators and Representative Larry Craig had attended NIBCA events in Coeur d'Alene over the years when I served as executive officer.

In 1988, Congressman Larry Craig, with support from Tom Foley, introduced the budget in the House of Representatives requesting partial funding of the two state Centennial Trail project. The amount requested would only fund about half of the estimated trail costs at that time, but it was approved. From the House, the trail funding was included in a bill to be reviewed by the Senate Appropriation Committee, Senator McClure was Chairman of that important committee.

At crunch time in the budget process, one of McClure's key staff called me in the Commissioner's office at the County, and asked if the funding for Washington's trail could be in this budget, and Idaho's in next years. I emphasized that it was a two-state trail project, and both states needed the funding in order to proceed. Thankfully, Senator McClure continued his support, and funding for both trails was included in the 1988-89 Federal budget which was signed by President Reagan. I was so pleased that the staff person who called me was someone I had previously met in the Senator's office.

This budget appropriation approved only about half of the amount needed by both states. Idaho received $1.35 million of an estimated $2.4 million to develop the Idaho trail. Washington received $3.4 million of their projected $5.9 million cost. The federal appropriation only covered trail construction and other costs such as land acquisition. Personnel, or equipment, had to be paid out of other funds. Other donation requests, and fund-raising events were scheduled to bring in the additional money needed. Local support was good and by 1989 The trail committee had commitments in excess of $250,000. Prospects looked good for raising the additional funds.

In the meantime, routing problems surfaced in Post Falls and along Seltice Way. Opposition to the trail surfaced in neighborhoods with people that started exhibiting the NIMBY syndrome (Not In My Back Yard). Some Post Falls residents seemed to feel that all

THE TRAIL THAT ALMOST WASN'T

the perverts from Spokane would be bicycling onto their part of the trail and make it unsafe. The Post Falls Highway District became upset when some of the mills expressed liability concerns about the trail interfering with some of their trucks.

People who had not expressed opposition to the trail when they believed it would not be built, came out strongly to oppose the trail at this strategic time. A letter was sent to Senator McClure by the Highway District in June of 1989, asking for the funding to be frozen because rights-of-way, and routing, was not properly secured and the trail organizers did not do due diligence when planning this unsafe routing project.

I was very upset at this action by the Post Falls Highway District because I felt the Committee had addressed these concerns during the planning process, and had looked at alternative routing and liability concerns. I felt because of pressure from others the Highway District had created false allegations concerning the trail planning process. I was personally very upset because of the admiration, and respect, I had for Senator McClure and how he must feel that I had misled him.

Even though the trail committee, and the cities of CDA and Post Falls still supported the trail routing, the controversy persisted, and Senator McClure asked for funds to be held up until the routing problems could be addressed. The County Commissioners invited the public to an informational meeting at North Idaho College held on August 10, 1989. County Commissioners Frank Henderson, and Bob Haakenson, sat on one side of the stage, while I sat with the trail committee on the other side of the stage. It seemed that about half of the 300 people in attendance supported the trail, and half didn't. I felt very upset at the hostility exhibited by some of the remarks that questioned the due diligence done by the trail committee. I felt personally responsible for some of the anger that was exhibited because I had helped get the support from Senator McClure. I felt very bad about the negative feelings expressed.

I resigned from the trail committee the day after that meeting because I did not want to be a "lightning rod" that would discourage support for the trail. The committee kindly asked me to continue, but I felt it would be better to work behind the scenes. I continued to support this Centennial project in many ways. I would like to state how much I admired the hard work done by Doug Eastwood, John Muller, and the rest of the Committee to work out Seltice routing problems.

One of the ways I helped was by concentrating on getting some State funds allocated toward the trail project. At a meeting in Coeur d'Alene, I approached Governor Andrus, and asked him if he couldn't help with some state funding. I could tell he wasn't aware of any funds that could be distributed for trails throughout the state, and I decided I would provide him with more information. From then on if I saw he was going to be in Coeur d'Alene, I would go to where he was, and hand him an update on our Centennial Trail and the need for State funding. I think he finally told one of his staff.... Please get that lady Commissioner off my back, and see if we can't find some funds to help with this trail.

We did eventually receive some money from one of the State funding sources for trails. I would like to add that Governor Andrus also became a strong supporter of the trail, and when we were raising funds by adding names to a monument in downtown CDA at Independence Point. Governor Andrus sent his personal

THE TRAIL THAT ALMOST WASN'T

check to me in the Commissioner's office so his name would be included.

The trail committee continued to work on routing between Post Falls and Coeur d'Alene, and also expressed strong interest in a trail section that might be possible east of Coeur d'Alene. I met with Rick Cummins, Superintendent for the north region of Idaho Parks and Recreation, and he said he could envision a pedestrian/bicycle route along one of the four abandoned Interstate lanes, when the new freeway was completed. This section of the Trail was in the County, and all three Commissioners supported that concept after I explained the possibilities of adding a beautiful five mile stretch along CDA Lake. It could be one of the most beautiful sections of the Trail, if it could be developed.

The ITD (Idaho Transportation Department), who had jurisdiction of that road until the new overpass was completed, was not excited about having the Centennial Trail on part of the abandoned highway. The Eastside Highway District wasn't too excited either. They were to take over that stretch of road after ITD had finished making improvements to a parking lot and boat launch by Higgins Point. Unfortunately, for the lake, in March 1990, a section of land near Higgins Point slid into the lake, and then another large area slipped into the lake in May, taking with it two pieces of earth moving equipment.

A lawsuit filed by the Kootenai Environment Alliance (KEA) by attorney Scott Reed cited violations of the Clean Water Act. The ITD had multiple problems with the permit, and fill material. Other state agencies began to sound the alarm that they too were not happy with the land slide and fill material that was polluting the lake. Although the Centennial Trail was not mentioned as a possible mitigation effort then, by late

1990 state representatives from northern Idaho and other parts of the state were calling upon ITD to extend the Trail along that scenic corridor. My special thanks to Scott Reed, who probably worked behind the scenes to make this happen.

So out of the mudslides came some beautiful lemonade for the trail committee. Yvonne Ferrell, Director of State Parks & Recreation, had become a trail supporter, and she welcomed the opportunity to have a pedestrian bicycle trail with enhancements of restrooms, and other amenities, under State Park jurisdiction. I had met Yvonne during my efforts to obtain some state funding, and she invited me to the dedication of that part of the Centennial Trail in 1995, which was after I had left the Commissioner's office. By then, most of the controversy over the Trail routing had been resolved, and people were beginning to realize what a wonderful legacy it will be for generations to come.

Improvements continued to made to the Trail system, even during the last decade. The Centennial Trail Foundation, and Committee worked with every opportunity to change a route and to make things safer and they succeeded in many places. A much better trail system thru the Riverstone properties was made possible by John Stone, developer of Riverstone.

Although working on the trail caused me a few heartaches, and several grey hairs, I am so proud of this lasting legacy for Idaho's Centennial. After I was unelected as a County Commissioner, I ended up moving to Spokane and was lucky to live across the Spokane River and a section of the trail near Avista off Mission Avenue. It was great to see so many people using the Washington section of the Trail.

When I moved back to Coeur d'Alene in 2001, I was fortunate enough to buy my dream home above the CDA

Lake Drive section of the Trail in the Silver Beach area. Every day, all year long, people are using, and enjoying the trail. There are many families and bicyclists and runners that I love watching them have fun. Most have smiles on their faces as they travel this very important Idaho Centennial legacy. I feel proud to have been a part of blazing this wonderful trail, and I am so thankful for Doug Eastwood, and the hard work of the Trail committee, who persevered for many years after Idaho's Centennial.

Out My Door
by Graham Christensen

    Ten thousand miles? I added up the time I've spent on the Centennial trail so far. At four to five days per week, and about four to five miles per day over the nine years we've lived on the Centennial Trail at Silver Beach, as best I can figure, I've averaged a thousand miles a year on the trail. Add six years in Coeur d'Alene before moving to Silver Beach, and I'm at ten thousand miles. Biking, running, triathlons, walking the dog, cruiser bikes with kids and friends, to Tony's or to town, teaching the kids to ride a bike, we've done it all.

    Living on the trail, we've used the trail in all seasons. The Centennial trail's ease of access, scenic beauty and connectivity draws all comers, all year round.

    In the winter, I pull out the fat bike, and ride in the snow, to Higgin's Point, dodging photographers, and salmon carcasses, along the way. Many days there are more photographers than eagles. Winter is my favorite time to run on the trail. With tights, gloves, a long sleeve and yak trax, I can get out on all but the wettest, and coldest, days and I can finish a decent run without losing five pounds of sweat. Short days mean most times on the trail are highlighted by a dramatic sunrise, or sunset, and then on some sunny February afternoons the trail clears of snow and I head out for a ride. There are still icicles on the cliffs but when the sun shines and the wind has died for the moment, you feel the early call of springtime, even through all my layers.

    Spring brings lonely training rides in the rain, getting ready for Ironman, or the next bike adventure I've always got on my calendar. March comes, and the frogs

THE TRAIL THAT ALMOST WASN'T

near Steamer's parking area cheer me through my next interval. Early season group rides follow the Centennial Trail to Washington, and the Rocket Bakery for pastries, cookies, and a mid-ride coffee. It's a vain attempt to achieve "race fitness" that always ends with plans for next season, when we will really take it seriously.

On sunny spring days, the trail seems to be at its busiest time. The parking lots fill up and it seems all of Coeur d'Alene is out enjoying the trail, ready to shake off the long dreary winter. Daylight savings comes, and it's time to pump up the tires on the dusty cruiser bikes for trips to town for dinners, and with friends that go too late. Who brought the lights this time?

In June, Ironman week always signals the official beginning of summer on the trail. There is so much anticipation, excitement, elation, and disappointment wrapped in one week. It's also the one week we get to show off the trail with the rest of the world. No matter whether you PR'd or DNF'd, at least you got to take in the views along the way.

In July and August, the weather warms and the best rides, and runs, in the summer finish with a dip in the lake. Getting back to the house after a long run, the kids can't tell if I've jumped in the lake or I'm just drenched in sweat. Summer's long days end in walks on the trail to friends' docks with a cooler of refreshments to watch another sunset over Tubbs Hill.

With August comes increasing thunderstorms. One afternoon we pulled out the cruiser bikes, and headed to Tony's for dinner. Sunshine turned to billowing clouds, and the threat of a storm. We quickly paid the bill, and left to a slight sprinkle which quickly turned to hail, and a downpour from the oncoming storm. We pedaled our hearts out, the kids laughing along the way, and pulled the bikes into the garage right as the first thunder boomed on the lake.

Fall is the best. September and October bring reasonable temperatures, access to beautiful forest roads, and earned fitness from a summer of activity. Rides start on the Centennial Trail but can end on Marie Saddle picking huckleberries, or with a boat shuttle home from Harrison, or Rockford Bay.

But some days are just nasty, and I don't want to go outside. On those days I look out the window, and there is always someone out there tougher, braver, stronger than me. No matter whether it is thirty-five and raining on slush or 100 degrees and smoky, there is always someone on the trail. Tomorrow, I tell myself, tomorrow I'll get back out there.

THE TRAIL THAT ALMOST WASN'T

I Want To Live Here
by Ivanka Kuran

I first came to Coeur d' Alene on a vacation in the summer of 2001. I remember staying at a hotel in town and being told there was a biking, and walking, trail that went to the end of the road at Higgens Point – the Centennial Trail. Being an avid biker, I thought I better check this out since this trail also went to the state line, and into Spokane. As I set off from downtown, I remember walking the trail along Lakeshore Drive and getting my first view of the Lake Coeur d'Alene by Silver Beach. I walked down to Tony's Restaurant, and enjoyed the benches, and bathrooms along the way, and the bikes I saw going past. The Centennial trail sold me **– I could live here!**

The next day I went in the opposite direction, adjacent to North Idaho College, out towards Post Falls, and I was impressed with the accessibility, and great condition of the trail. Later that year, I moved to Coeur d'Alene, that's when my love affair with the Centennial Trail began – biking, and running, on the trail each week.

In 2003, Ironman CDA came to town, and the marathon piece was all along the trail. So many miles, and stories, along the Centennial Trail as I did 13 Ironman races. I practically know each post by name! The Bennett Bay Hill has been the site of many hill repeats. I have shared the miles with so many friends, enjoying the hours, and places, the trail led us. Favorite days are early morning, or in colder weather, when it seems I have the trail all to myself. The views, and condition, of the Centennial trail is unparalleled, and I think how lucky I am to live here, and near this amazing resource. I am grateful for the continued vision of the trail committee in incorporating the trail's use in new developments, as the city continues to grow.

As the years have gone by, my love affair with the Centennial Trail continues – I moved to be closer to this amazing connector. I have seen the sponsorships, and support, of the trail grow – as has its usage with families, and retirees, enjoying the wide path. I consider myself fortunate to live in a community that supports an active lifestyle. I enjoy and use the trail every week and it has woven its way into my life – like a good friend waiting to share in my latest bike ride or walk. Thank you for the years of happy "adventures" on the amazing Centennial Trail!

THE TRAIL THAT ALMOST WASN'T

A Memorial Run
by Jennie Lamb

Many years ago, a friend and I were participating in the Spring Dash, the five-mile race that kicks off the running season as well as raises money for local causes.
It's a sweet little race that includes a "Tot Trot" for really little runners as well as being, prior to Covid, and virtual races, a qualifier for Bloomsbury Second Seedings.
Part of the Spring Dash route is along the Centennial Trail.

So, on this beautiful sunny spring day, the kind we would refer to as a bluebird day if we had skis on rather than running shoes, my friend, and I, were jogging along the trail. We are not "real runners, " so it was more like jog for a mile or two, then walk, repeat.
It was during a walk cycle when we met the man. He was obviously much more of a runner than us, but for some reason he too was walking.

We struck up a conversation and learned that this gentleman had made a commitment to himself to run a race in every one of the 50 states. He wasn't a professional runner, just a regular kind of guy.

He was doing this as a tribute to his wife. I wish I remembered his name, or the specific details of his story, but I do remember the emotions it stirred in me. He, and his bride, had been married a long time when she had been diagnosed with a life-threatening illness. The challenge to run a race in every state was how he grieved.

In writing this, I googled "man who runs in all 50 states," thinking I might put a name to the man. I learned of many men who are doing similar challenges and a few who, like this man, are doing it in memory of a loved one.

The man shared this story. He shared while walking the Centennial Trail along our beautiful lake on a bluebird kind of day.

You just never know who you're gonna meet...

Growing Up On The Trail
by Jenny Wayman

Happy 30th anniversary to the North Idaho Centennial Trail! Quite an accomplishment on the part of some future-sighted residents.

So, the trail is now the age of my now adult daughter, who as soon as she was strong enough to sit up in the seat of the bike trailer, and see from underneath her bike helmet, she enjoyed rides with her big brother to, and from, City Park, from our Garden District home downtown.

As the years flew by, the trail was a safe place for our kids to ride, without the fear of busy traffic. The trail was a piece of independence for young riders, and security for their mothers. Who doesn't remember the thrill of riding your bike and cruising?

The trail elicits a feeling of gratitude for the dreamers and creators. A sense of respect for the many hours of work by an army of community members who created a fun place for so many, for many years.

The trail is quiet much of the time, with the site of water on a hot summer day, while at other times it is a ribbon of activity winding through our beautiful town.

This trail, meandering through our parks, and along our river, calls to all of us to come out and play and share the good feeling with others in our community.

One of my favorite remembrances of riding the Centennial Trail is Mothers' Day of 2007. My son, Jake, invited me on a "special outing" he had planned. We were to ride the Centennial Trail ALL the way from Coeur d'Alene to Post Falls. Just the two of us! He was excited and I was touched.

At nine years old, he had enough money saved to treat me to lunch at the Post Falls Jack in the Box. Jake felt so grown up; I felt so honored.

The trail provided a true adventure, in that it seemed like a significant journey- yet quite a reasonable idea for a young kid to conceive of taking.

This Mothers' Day celebration of a boy and his mother, enjoying a bike ride together, lasted many years. And when Jake was an adult living in Utah, and then Virginia, he would still reference his wish that we were riding the trail together again on Mothers' Day, "just like we always did."

Always Close To The Trail
by Joe Abate

When my wife Kathi and I moved to Coeur d'Alene in 2001, we were delighted by the wide supply of bicycle trails – the Trail of the Coeur d'Alene's, the Hiawatha Trail, and especially the North Idaho Centennial Trail. In those days, the Trail was relatively new, and not heavily used.

We lived in a house on top of Blackwell Hill, and while it was easy for me to ride into town, it was not easy, or desirable, for my two young children to ride their bicycles across U.S. Highway 95, or across the bridge spanning the Spokane River coming into Coeur d'Alene.

In 2005, we rented our home to several triathletes from Austin, Texas, and moved into the small apartment above the house while we watched them prepare for the big race. We were invited to join the competitors, and their spouses, for dinner one night where we met all the participants, and they shared their stories. Our children were excited to be a part of the Ironman event. They made posters with the Texas athletes' names on them, and sat on the side of the road on U.S. 95 to cheer them on, beginning a relationship that has lasted to this day.

In the early Ironman years, I volunteered in the medical tent and tended to the triathletes who had gone beyond the limits of their bodies, some after they had crossed the finish line and some, unfortunately, before they could finish the race. I would often ride my bike on the Ironman route as well as the CDA Triathlon route, both of which included portions of the Centennial Trail.

We moved several times during our time in Coeur d'Alene. Each time, our decision was to live someplace that had easy access to the Centennial Trail. After years of protected riding away from downtown traffic, I had no desire to be far from the trail that offered me a chance to get my mileage in while avoiding the vagaries of busy auto traffic.

We moved from Blackwell Hill to the Fort Grounds in 2008, where our house was only one block away from the Centennial Trail, accessed via the portion of the trail that ran along the edge of the North Idaho College campus and behind the water treatment facility. From this location, everyone in the family had easy access to the trail, and could ride to the lake, The Coeur d'Alene Resort, and downtown, or head north along the river to Riverstone, soccer fields, the church, and The Kroc Center.

For years, our children lived the true lake life, riding their bikes everywhere, enjoying the beach, Fort Sherman Playground, and the lake. I rode the trail as often as I could, enjoying the incredible scenery out past the Coeur d'Alene Resort Golf Course, past Michael D's, onto Coeur d'Alene Lake Drive, and along the lakefront to Higgens Point, where a climb up the hill led to a beautiful scenic viewpoint at the top.

In 2009, when our children attended Gonzaga Prep, they and several of their friends decided to celebrate the last day of school by riding from Spokane back to Coeur d'Alene. I accompanied them as they rode over 20 miles on the Centennial Trail.

We moved to a condominium at Riverstone in 2015, and our patio looked directly out onto the trail. We were able to see all the traffic leading to downtown. It was astonishing how busy the trail had become over the years since we first came to town. One of our favorite memories was on the fourth of July, watching the steady stream of bicycle lights as they wound their way home in the dark following the fireworks. Each year, the procession would last for over an hour.

THE TRAIL THAT ALMOST WASN'T

In 2016, Bike to Work Week was held from June 6-10. I was working at Heritage Health at the time, and we decided to promote the event among our staff, encouraging the willing, and able, to ride their bikes for a week rather than use their automobiles. It didn't seem right to encourage others to do it if I did not, so I rode every day that week, and enjoyed it so much, I decided to declare a personal Bike to Work Year. It was an unusually mild winter that year in the city and I was able to ride for an entire year, with the exception of approximately three weeks that the trail was too icy or covered with snow. With proper clothing and a good set of fenders, it never seemed too cold, or too wet, to consider the trip, although there was a day or two so cold that shifting was difficult because the cables were stuck, or the derailleur grease was too thick to shift smoothly.

I rode from home to office, office to clinic, back to the office, and back home most days, the majority of which was on the Centennial Trail. The longest day was when I needed to visit our Post Falls office. Luckily the weather was warm, and sunny, and I had the time to make the trip without interfering with the rest of the workday. Once again, almost the entire trip was by way of the Centennial Trail.

I often kept track of my mileage using MapMyRide, but it really wasn't about the mileage. What I noticed most was how much better I felt starting the day with a bike ride rather than a car ride, and how each day started with more energy, a clearer mind, and a great deal more peace. Over the year, I came to realize I had discovered the antidote to the stress, and anxiety, that accompanied a busy cardiologist's work schedule, and the somewhat toxic American culture. At that point, tracking the miles was meaningless.

In 2016, I had to bring my parents from Sun City West to Coeur d'Alene because of their health issue. They lived in an assisted living facility in Post Falls for two years, then moved to another facility on Kathleen Ave. Just over the fence in the backyard of that facility lies the Centennial Trail, so I could easily ride my bike to visit them. I also liked to walk the trail with my dad, a vigorous walker, even at age 95, he would walk the Trail for two miles to The Kroc Center and back. This continued until the 2020 pandemic, when he was forced to abandon the Trail and avoid contact with others.

One winter, we had a snowstorm that snarled traffic and prevented bike travel. Kathi and I put on our cross-country skis and skied from the front door of the condo to the assisted living facility to see Mom and Dad.

After just a couple of years, we sold the condo at Riverside and bought a new home near Atlas and Hanley. Once again, one of our main criteria was easy access to the Centennial Trail, which is only a block away.

I retired in 2018, and during the pandemic I was offered a job at the Trek bike store in Coeur d'Alene. I jumped at the chance to end my social isolation. As an essential service (transportation), the bike store was a great place to meet new people, and see old friends, some of whom I had not seen in five years or more. I am delighted to share the joy of cycling with others, and when out of town visitors ask for suggestions on where to ride, I gladly point to the stack of maps we keep in the shop – maps of the Centennial Trail.

It Started in Billings
By Jonathan Mueller, FASLA, PLA

The earliest discussions of a regional trail system came in late 1986, or early 1987, when I was helping Doug Eastwood with an update to the City of Coeur d'Alene's park system plan. I was serving on the Parks & Recreation Commission and in those days the city had no money to hire the specialty consultants necessary to do such a plan. So, the work was completed as an internal project with volunteers.

When the document was finished, Doug asked me, "Have we missed anything?" I answered that the only thing not really discussed was the need, and benefit, of a city-wide, or regional trail system, as both linear park and an agent of connectivity. Doug wanted to know more about the basis for this and I related my recent experience in Montana while working for Ted Wirth's organization in Billings, Montana.

I had been part of a large interdisciplinary team of consultants that planned, designed and oversaw the construction of what basically was a new city on the plains of southeast Montana. The Colstrip project was developed and completed in support of energy development, which in the late 1970s and early 1980s, was a big deal. Ted called it an 'energy newtown'. Newtown being a fashionable term of that era. Basically, the team was taking a city of 1,500, or so residents, and growing it to a peak of 12,500 people at the height of construction, and then planning for a managed transition to a stable population of around 7,500.

As landscape architects working on the project, we engaged in ongoing planning, design and construction oversight, working side-by-side with architects, and engineers, on behalf of the consortium of power companies that were constructing not only the expanded city, but also Colstrip power plants 3 and 4. It was a significant effort as all the components of a city had to be built, both above ground, and below ground. Gray and green infrastructure were developed on a parallel track along with quality living facilities as was necessary to ensure human health, and well-being of the future residents.

One of the significant aspects of the larger project became the development of a separated, and paved, Class 1 bike trail along the major arterials of the new city. The trail also linked the new city to the old city. The urban trail ultimately wound its way throughout the community. It was advocated by a landscape architect by the name of David Groshens, and by the time I left Montana to return to Coeur d'Alene, it was pretty much completed. It linked all the parks, schools, neighborhoods, and the main commercial, and civic areas of the town. It was very well used. Having had the chance to design, and build, a portion of this spine, to see its use, impact, and value to a park system tickled the imagination of what could emerge in Coeur d'Alene and the larger community. It was an exciting prospect that could take shape locally.

At that time, Doug had a lot on his plate with pending new parks, the need for establishment of funding mechanisms and the maintenance of what the city already had. He said he liked the idea and would include it as a larger aspiration, but would take it up in more detail when he cleared the deck of the more pressing near-term issues he faced.

It wasn't long after that when I got a call from Doug. He said, "I think we have an opportunity to now look at your notion of a city-wide trail system. Only this opportunity may be much larger in scale to include the whole county." He went on to explain that he had been contacted by officials from Spokane City, and Spokane County, about the possibility of a two-state trail system running from Spokane to Coeur d'Alene along the Spokane River corridor. The projects were envisioned to be part of the centennial celebrations for both Washington, and Idaho, to occur in 1989 and 1990, respectively. With the larger concept of a trail system as part of the aspirations of a council-adopted park system plan, the basis to go forward with the project, as a matter of policy, was already established.

And so, the effort began, and as we all know offered many challenges in getting to that first use...and expanded in scope to include the piece from east Sherman to Higgins Point on the lake.

In the 30 years since the initial phases opened, the trail has continued to be used, improved upon and expanded as we had envisioned in the original master plan. Both linear park and major element of regional connectivity, we indeed have the lasting-legacy, as originally envisioned, one that continues to get better and better. The only aspect to the original vision not fully developed is the telling of the cultural/natural history of the river corridor. It has such a rich history and many stories to tell. My hope is that we can more fully take that next step to better present and ultimately tell the story of this place we call home---'In all the west, no spot like this!'

My First Triathlon
by Laura Sferra

In 2015, I started training for my first triathlon, and it began on the Centennial Trail. As a new runner, and cyclist, the trail was a safe and friendly place to start. Its travelers often greet you with a smile, or a wave, and it has been a great gathering place for active people to support one another. Over the past six years, I have continued to challenge myself on the trail as I prepared for the half Ironman, and full Ironman races. Whether I am biking or running, it is where I can push myself and redefine my limits.

The Centennial Trail has also been my place to go to gather my thoughts, and to connect with myself. I often pause to appreciate the sounds of birds singing, the waves of the lake crashing on the shore, and the view of the mountain ranges. Every season brings new adventures and beauty. The scenery along the trail is soothing, and it is often where I can release stress, and find a sense of calm.

My Wheelchair and The Trail
by Lloyd Stewart

The main reason Lloyd Stewart and his wife, Gracie, purchased their home in Riverstone was so that he could wheel out his front door, and onto the Centennial Trail.

When Lloyd was 19, he lost his left leg in an industrial accident. He worked for a prosthetic limb business in Seattle, ultimately purchased, and owned, it for 17 years - until surgery forced him to retire.

Lloyd and Gracie had family in Northern Idaho, and in 1986 decided to return to Sandpoint, where Gracie had grown up. They bought a 148-acre farm in Samuels, north of Sandpoint, with pasture, and forest that they hired people to log. Gracie also worked as a substitute teacher, and volunteered in schools.

Lloyd frequently drove to Coeur d'Alene for medical appointments; diabetes was also a factor in his life. After many years, they decided to move closer to medical care, sold the farm, and bought a house in Dalton Gardens, just north of Coeur d'Alene. Lloyd was still walking at this time.

During their years in Dalton Gardens, Lloyd's health dwindled, and he was forced to use a wheelchair. Without sidewalks, Dalton Gardens was not conducive to wheelchairs, so he and Gracie would drive to Riverstone Park and traverse the trail around the pond. On one of those trips, they noticed houses under construction next to the Centennial Trail, and bought a lot for a new house. They moved into the house in 2016, and "have never looked back."

In the summer months, Lloyd, often accompanied by Gracie and their Maltese, Rose, wheeled many miles on the trail, a minimum of twice each day. Even in rainy weather, "I am ready, and raring to go." In the winter, he gets out at least once.

Their distance varies. Lloyd and Gracie also have mobility scooters with a 30-mile range. They travel on the trail to the north side of I-90, as far as Kathleen, and to the University of Idaho building on the banks of the Spokane River, or to the baseball field by The Kroc Center for picnics amongst the shade trees. They love the waterfront area by Le Peep, and often travel south as far as City Park. Covid and the crowds have recently kept them from circumventing the lake in Riverstone Park.

Lloyd appreciates that the trail is plowed in winter, finds most cyclists to be very respectful of wheelchairs, and loves sharing the trail with Rose, who hops into Lloyd's lap when she's gone far enough.
Exercise is critical for Lloyd, with his diabetes, and confinement to a wheelchair. "The trail is a lifesaver for more than one reason. Just the peace of mind, the serenity of it. Living here has worked out extremely well."

And that seemed like the end of the story, but the next chapter is just unfolding. In February of 2021, Lloyd, Gracie and Rose moved to a ninth-floor condominium in One Lakeside, across from City Park. With only Northwest Boulevard between them and Lake Coeur d'Alene, the Centennial Trail is still a central part of their lives, and allows them to easily wheel to McEuen Park, City Park, the dike road and more.

Once again, Lloyd said, "It's working out extremely well."

It Became Our Lifeline
by Ruth Pratt

The Centennial Trail (C.T.) has long been a focal point of attraction in our lives. Now in our senior years, my husband and I support, defend, and use the trail regularly, in all seasons. We even chose the site of our retirement house (in the Riverstone area) based on its proximity to the Trail. Like us, the Trail has seen many things during its existence: boards, bikes, scooters, wheelchairs, dogs, skates, and countless feet running, walking, skipping, hopping, and dancing. But (also like us,) it has never witnessed a global pandemic. In this past year of "unprecedented", "unknowns", and "uncertainties", the Trail took on a new dimension in our lives: constant companion, safe refuge, and connection with the outside world during isolation. It did, in fact, become our lifeline!

Almost every day starting in March of 2020, and progressing through four subsequent seasons, we walked out the back gate of our neighborhood, and the Trail was there to greet us with open arms. That embrace was so welcoming, regardless of the weather... coaxing us out of our small bubble to explore the natural world. All we had to do was decide whether to walk east, or west, to be reminded that nature, at least, was still there for us. Inside, watching the news of an evolving pandemic and changing guidelines about what was safe, we seemed to be holding our breath in anticipation of the next scary turn of events. Outside, thanks to the Trail, we were able to breathe fresh air (mask-filtered) and reacquaint ourselves with the constancy of the natural world.

Because our "home stretch" of the Trail runs along the Spokane River, and adjacent to two parks

(Riverstone and Atlas), we encountered a full spectrum of flora and fauna with the changing seasons. Ducks were our most prevalent companions...mallards, buffleheads, and the occasional merganser flew, tipped, dove, and went about their normal routines. They brought a sense of constancy amid turmoil. Herons, eagles, geese, and osprey reminded us that the patterns of their lives, at least, remained unchanged. The abundance of plants and trees, both new and old, as well as the beautiful landscaping that emerged in the new Atlas Park, responded to the seasonal changes, and brought us joy.

But the most precious gift the Trail gave us was the opportunity to interact with other people (and their many dogs of all sizes and varieties) who came out in record numbers for exercise and interaction (albeit at a distance). We learned to recognize friends in masks by the smile in their eyes and the sound of their muffled voices. We could stop and visit and feel hopeful that things were moving forward toward something safer. In other words, the Trail gave us hope, and reassurance, over this past weird year.

I realize that I am personifying things here, but when we assign human characteristics to nonhuman entities, we are deciding what is worthy of our time and care. Truly, the Trail deserves that, and so much more for the role it plays in our lives. It deserves a love song!

Involved From the Beginning
by Sandy Emerson

Doug Eastwood, city of Coeur d'Alene Parks Director, and I were well-acquainted, when I was at the Coeur d'Alene Area Chamber as the Executive Director in 1980-1987. We had previously worked on waterfront and other city projects. I was aware of efforts in Washington to create an extend public trail corridor from Spokane to the state line on the Washington side. The idea was to continue the trail from the state line across North Idaho to Coeur d'Alene, and possibly beyond. Randy Haddock and Evelyn Adams, key members of the Trail Committee and its foundation also were, and are, friends. I respect and value their input, dedication, and participation, as I do Doug's persistence and enthusiasm for whatever it is that he does.

Doug made me aware of the road blocks the sawmills had become in having the trail along Seltice Way where the "Old Highway," as I-90/US-10 was known then, ran as a divided federal transcontinental route. This road was part of the interstate highway system from Seattle to Chicago and on across the country when I was a boy, before the I-90 Interstate Highway – "the freeway" – was completed. Opened in 1960 or so, it relegated the old highway, now Seltice Way, to a local access" back" road to Post Falls. As a local access two-lane boulevard, it seemed logical to Doug, the committee, and others, including me, that this was the natural place for the trail to be. It could run alongside the old highway, in the wide shoulder right-of-way, especially given its now significantly reduced traffic flow.

Doug knew I had worked closely on numerous community projects, and civic programs with the sawmill owners such at Idaho Forest Industries (IFI) and local managers and operators of Central Premix., a Spokane-based company. These companies were next door to each other along the south side of Seltice Way coming into Northwest Boulevard, the major west side entrance to the city. These owners and managers balked at having the trail follow the old highway in front of their long-established, busy industrial operations.

I agreed to contact the owner and president of IFI, Tom Richards, and Cliff Anderson, manager of Central Premix about gaining their cooperation. Both were, and still are, long-time friends, even family friends for generations in the case of the Richards connection. While their receptions were friendly, and remained cordial, even after learning I was there to support the case for the trail location along the road right-of-way in front of their businesses. Both in turn, explained the liability in their eyes was far too great, with dozens of logging trucks, and cement trucks, coming and going from the access roads into their businesses, sometimes hourly during busiest times of the year – the same good days for users of the trail. They told me there could be hundreds, or more, of daily trips by loaded, and hightailing empty trucks, running to and from those businesses. Visibility of walkers and bikes from the big rigs would be an issue as well, they pointed out.

These long-time community supporters could not see their way to accept the danger to their companies, or to the trail users. Thanking them for listening to me after having had the same pleas a number of times before, I reported back to Doug, and Evalyn, my futile efforts. The trail eventually ended up along the highway right-of-Way in this stretch, not a bad accommodation, thanks to the good folks at the Idaho Department of Transportation, who, it turns out, have a soft spot for moving people on bicycles, and people walking, to safely get the pedestrians across, and along, their roads and highways.

The annotation to this story is that a few years later, when the Trail Foundation initiated the "Adopt-a-Trail" program, I was again contacted by still involved trail volunteer, Randy Haddock. He asked me if the Sunrise Rotary Club would like to adopt a mile of the trail for a trail clean -up program. I asked if we could have a part of the trail along Seltice Way, which was arranged, and the board approved it. Twenty years later, club members still participate in Trail cleanup days in the spring, and before major holidays. Artwork has been added. Sailboats at the park and trail parking lot by the intersection of Seltice Way, Ironwood Drive, and Northwest Boulevard along the same stretch of the old Highway in front of what was the sawmill and the cement plant. In the trailhead park, where the club members gather for the cleanup by the Sailboats art feature, is also found a granite slab turned into an interesting bench seat in the form of a spider – "A-rock-nid", it's called and continues to be a joy each time we take a walk along this amazing public trail, "The Trail That Almost Wasn't," as Doug's book title calls it, and those who were there would agree.

Historic plaques and interpretive signs about areas of interest continue to be added along the route of the trail, helping to make it an attraction to be enjoyed every time we use the trail, while getting fresh air and healthy exercise.

In Our Retirement
by Tere Porcarelli

For so many years, while working in Coeur d'Alene, my husband, Steve McCrea and I, often cycled in the early morning into the sunrise, and after-work rides back into the sunset. We enjoyed each ride, and each was different from every other. The weather, the season, and of course, the proverbial tail wind as we would be flying effortlessly until we rounded back from Higgins Point towards town and chuckled, "It got us again".

Now in our retirement, we ride more during daytime hours and meet walkers, runners, and riders on a variety of human powered, and electric, bicycles from all over our country, enjoying our precious Centennial Trail.

In our running days, there was nothing better than running Tubbs Hill, and extending the run onto the Centennial Trail along the east shore of the lake.

We never take for granted how lucky we are to have the Centennial Trail to ride to the Rocket Cafe (The Rocket Ride) and enjoy a treat with coffee, and ride back to Coeur d'Alene.

An Amazing Discovery
by Tim Keaty

After being around all the Ironman races, and triathlons, in North Idaho, I decided I would do one for myself. So, I signed up for the Hayden Sprint Triathlon and started training.

The Prairie Trail, a spur of the North Idaho Centennial trail is not too far away from my home. I thought it would make for a nice little ride, but I really had no idea where the Prairie Trail was, or if it really existed. I must have heard something about it being "off Huetter" or "in that general area." But, even if I didn't find the trailhead, or if it was not worth riding, I could always stay on the surface roads, avoid traffic, and eventually make my way back home. I still needed to complete a workout ride.

After retrieving my 20-year-old mountain bike, and pumping up the tires, I started out to find the trail. Riding a few miles west from the Hayden area and south on Huetter, I came to the Prairie Trailhead. I really had no idea what I'd find, but when I did, it was an obvious, and inviting starting point. Come to think of it, it was not even that far away from my home.

Immediately upon entering the trail, I noticed my bike tires purring along on smoothly paved asphalt. They almost made a melodious humming sound with an old song which I just could not quite pull up out of my memories. There was plenty of room for me and the others walking their dogs, in-line skating and what not. Signs told me exactly where I was, and how far to the next landmark.

The next things I noticed, as I intersected with the Centennial Trail, was how remarkably well-kept the trail was, and the beautiful scenery. Traveling south I went in, and out of, "Hobo Junction," the section of the trail that runs right along the wide beginning of the Spokane river, then into Riverstone, and on to North Idaho College. Along the college dike road there were all types of people on the beach enjoying a spring day, seemingly without a care in the world. Then I had an "Aha!" moment and I literally said to myself, "What a wonderful place to live. All this from a trail not far from my front door!" And I added, "Wow! They did this trail right." I was so impressed.

When one has a typical interaction with an employee at a retail store, trying on shoes, or a customer service call with an internet provider, rarely does one give it much more thought. When it's over, it's over and it's forgotten. Certainly, we won't bring it up in conversation, unless it is exceptionally good or remarkably poor.

After my first ride, I found myself telling everyone I had occasion to chat with about this great trail system. "Have you ever ridden on it? Are you aware we have this really beautiful trail going through town? Do you know how long it has been there?" These comments were all part of my conversation with just about everyone I spoke with.

One person I spoke with was as eager to talk about it as me. She responded with, "Yes, I know all about the Centennial Trail, and I have ridden the whole thing, all 23 miles."

I replied, "What? 23 miles? It doesn't go that far, does it?" Then she said she rides it to work sometimes, and that the trail has been here as long as she has lived here. Turns out she was on the board of the North Idaho Centennial Trail Foundation. After I shared how impressed I was that the cities, and county, would make a trail like this, she told me something incredible: "It's the citizens who have the responsibility to take care of, maintain, promote and expand the trail. The City of Post Falls, Kootenai County, and the City of Coeur d'Alene do a lot, but it is not part of their tax revenue plan to repair, manage and do upkeep. They do a lot and we could not take care of it without them, but we, the users, and citizens, need to take some responsibility for the long-term care of this trail."

A year or two later, I found myself sitting happily on the North Idaho Centennial Trail Board, involved in all things trail related.

I recently rode the same course that I first took when I "discovered" the Centennial Trail. As I finished my ride, I started thinking about how many times and how many miles I had been on the trail. I tried to do some quick calculations in my head; 50-60 times out and back along Lakeshore Drive to Higgens Point, Saturday morning rides out past Stateline, and The Prairie Trail to North Idaho College. The calculations quickly went beyond my ability to hold all the numbers or to keep a running tab in my head. There was no way I could account for all the miles. Hundreds of miles. Riding, running, getting out along Lake Coeur d'Alene, or the Spokane River, walking along, and crossing the trail to get to the transition area to start the ride portion of a triathlon. My wife and I ride our tandem bike, and walk the dike road to find a cozy spot to enjoy the afternoon. Running, riding, listening to music or having a beer at "Ales for the Trail" or at "Live after Five" in McEuen Park. As I continued to catalogue my trail use, it seemed like wherever I went and whatever I did, the trail was part of it.

Then, thankfulness. I could not help but be thankful that the trail has been available to me, to my family and friends anytime day or night, not far from my front door. These thoughts were followed by a twinge of obligation to send a check to support the trail. I figure I should support it. Then gratitude. I am glad to give a little of my time, talent, and resources to support the trail for the people of our community. I hope you'll join me and do the same.

A Big Part of His Recovery
by Tony Malaghan and Astrid Rial

In August 2014, Tony and Astrid Malaghan, and their son, Ronan, moved to Coeur d'Alene from Lakewood, Washington to improve their quality of life, including non-motorized transportation as part of their daily activities. They bought a house in downtown Coeur d'Alene so they could be close to the Centennial Trail.

Four years later, Tony had a freak accident that injured his carotid artery, and caused a massive stroke. Tony experienced significant right-side physical impairments, but one year later he got "back in the saddle" and started using the trail regularly again. You can spot him around town on his CAT trike that is equipped with a motor.

We use the trail for transportation and exercise. From our house, we ride to Higgens Point for a vigorous ride up the hills, ride downtown to go to the library, a pub or restaurant, and ride along the river to enjoy the cool breeze off of Lake Coeur d'Alene.

Since Tony is not driving a vehicle yet, riding on the trail gives him "transportation independence." In addition to bicycle riding, Astrid also uses the trail almost daily to walk their dog, Bundie. And, except for in the winter, we rarely drive downtown since parking a bicycle is much easier than parking a car. Getting back on a bike after the stroke has been very important for Tony's well-being. If we lived in a place where a bike trail was not accessible, Tony would feel homebound. Instead, he gets out in the community and is returning to the places and activities he enjoys.

We regularly travel the entire trail. All of our family enjoys the changing scenery during each season, enjoying that we can ride 15-20 miles without having to drive the bikes to a trail.

Keep up the great work in maintaining the trail. We appreciate it!

Epilogue

An Everlasting Legacy

The North Idaho Centennial Trail is recognized today as a landmark outdoor recreation facility. A recent study indicated that over 400,000 people use the trail every year. Since the trail was completed, steady improvements have been generated, making it better and safer along the 23-mile linear corridor. A recent economic impact study confirmed that the Centennial Trail is a strong economic engine for the community.

Early opposition to the trail routing has been turned into support of the trail. People who opposed the trail in the early days now express their appreciation for the trail, use it frequently, and feel it enhances their quality of life.

The North Idaho Centennial Trail has become the connecting point for trails through-out the community. The Prairie Trail, the Atlas Trail and soon the Highway 41 trail, are examples of Centennial Trail connections. The Idaho Transportation Department is rebuilding the U.S. 95 Trail and extending it to the Northern border of Kootenai County. Someday, this trail will connect Coeur d'Alene to Sandpoint. There are multiple access points to the North Idaho Centennial Trail from nearly anywhere along the 23-mile route. Find a listing of parking places for the trail at the end of this book.

Since the debate over the use of the Seltice Way Corridor, Coeur d'Alene has annexed that road all the way to Huetter. They have installed two pedestrian and bike paths on both sides of the corridor, similar to what was proposed originally, so many years ago. The continuation of that work should be considered by the

PFHD to extend a class I trail along Seltice way from Huetter to Highway 41. The right of way is plenty wide to accommodate the ever-increasing use and need for this trail.

Chapter 1 identified the different classes of trail development, classes I, II, and III. The North Idaho Centennial Trail, when first developed had 15 miles of class I trail, 7 miles of class II trail and one mile of class III trail. Steady improvements over the years now shows the North Idaho Centennial Trail to have 19 miles of class I trail and 4 miles of class II trail. The one mile stretch of the least preferred class III trail has been upgraded and converted to class II.

Trail width has evolved over the years since the trail was first installed. The first pedestrian/bicycle path in the area was the paved trail along the east side of Highway 95. That trail was eight feet in width. The problem with that width is when two people walking side by side in one direction encountered two other people walking side by side in the opposite direction, there was not enough room to pass each other without someone stepping off the trail. That problem was compounded when bicycles, people pushing strollers and dog walkers were added onto the trail use. An eight-foot-wide trail was determined to be too narrow for a community that would be growing in population and seeing increased use on the proposed Centennial Trail.

Early in the planning stages the trail committee and architect determined the Centennial Trail could not be any narrower than 10 feet. This was extremely problematic wherever a class II trail would be necessary. There was inevitably not enough room in the road right-of-way to accommodate 10 more feet for pedestrians and bicyclists. This was even more true, if a class II trail was proposed for both sides of the street. More discussion and long-term expectations led the trail committee to recommend a width of no less than 12 feet for new trails with an emphasis of working towards class I trails wherever possible. Class II trails, in roadways, are still narrow. Most class II widths are averaging about five or six feet in width.

By 2005 the county population was growing rapidly. The recommendation being put forward was to construct class I trails at a width between 14 to 16 feet. The North Idaho Centennial Trail is fortunate to have that width on most of its class I development.

Adversity that hovered over the trail project 30 years ago has long disappeared. The City of Coeur d'Alene, City of Post Falls, Kootenai County, Idaho State Parks and Recreation and the North Idaho Centennial Trail Foundation continue to work closely together to keep this trail the legacy that it is.

We are fortunate to have some of the best outdoor trails in the country. The U.S. Highway 95 trail is being rebuilt and widened. The subsequent development of the Hiawatha Trail and the Trail of The Coeur d'Alene's combined with the North Idaho Centennial Trail and Spokane River Centennial Trail make this area a paradise for walkers, runners, and bicycle enthusiasts.

The North Idaho Centennial Trail belongs to you, the people. It took a long time to build and it did not come easy. Thank you for all the support you have provided to ensure the success of this legacy trail.

Points of Interest
Along the North Idaho Centennial Trail

The 23-mile Centennial Trail provides a wealth of history and interest along its corridor: You will come across restaurants, bakeries, hotels, gift shops, bike shops, coffee shops and breweries...a little something for everyone, of every age, to enjoy. Your adventure is just beginning.

A Quick Response Code (QRC) at the end of this chapter will allow you to download the entire trail map for your convenience. The QRC map includes both the North Idaho Centennial Trail and the Spokane River Centennial Trail.

The following pages illustrate historic landmarks and places of interest. The journey begins at the Idaho/Washington state line and travels eastward toward Coeur d'Alene and ends at Higgins Point; Mile 23.

The North Idaho Centennial Trail Bridge

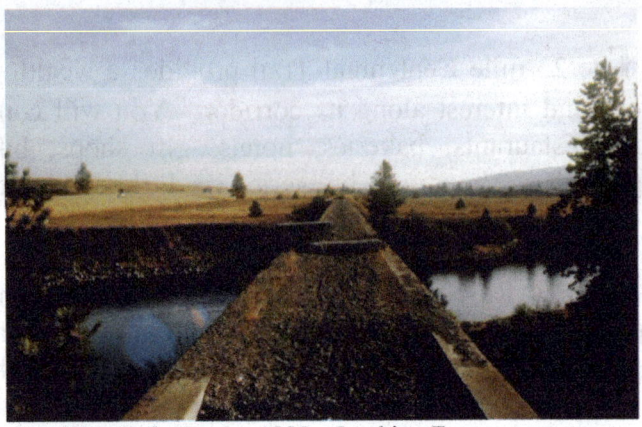

Photo by CDA Parks Dept – 1988 – Looking East

Built in 1910 by the Old Milwaukee Railroad, this bridge now serves as the scenic connection to the Idaho and Washington trails. The restored bridge is over 300 feet in length. Northern and southern views from the bridge are spectacular any time of the year as the Spokane River continues its journey westward.

The historic railroad bridge was rebuilt and opened for pedestrian use in October 1990. It was refurbished in 2017.

A trail head parking lot can be accessed at Exit 299 from I-90 in Washington. The lot is located on the corner of Spokane Bridge St. and Appleway Blvd. The bridge is approximately ¼ mile east of the parking lot.

Commemorative 40-Ton Boulder at the state line

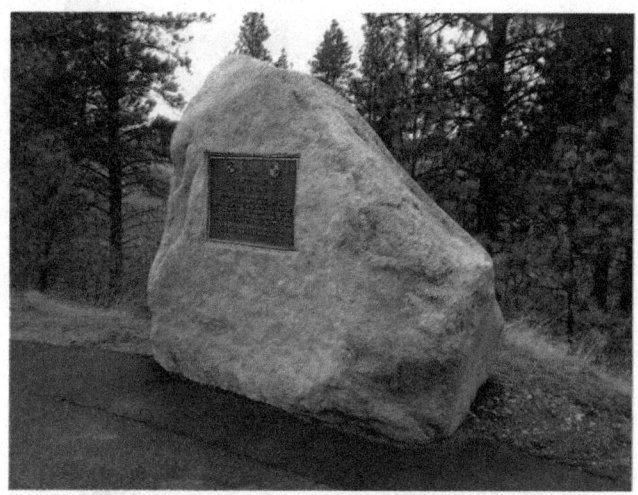

Photo by CDA Parks Dept

This boulder was put in place approximately 100 feet west of the historic railroad bridge and marks the line separating Idaho and Washington. The Idaho and Washington Surveyor Associations re-surveyed and confirmed the state line during trail development based on data from the 1800's. Central Pre-Mix Concrete Company donated the massive rock. A bronze plaque is set into a carved-out area of the rock commemorating the trail accomplishment.

Aquafer Drinking Water Hand Pump

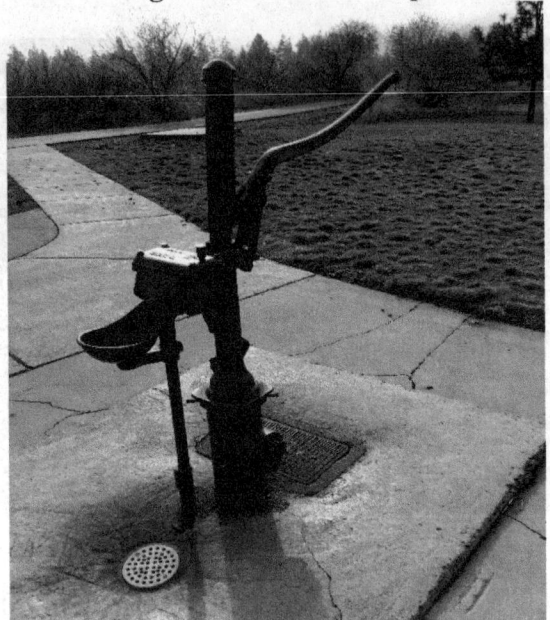

Photo by Kootenai County Parks Dept

This drinking fountain is located about 1/10 of a mile east of the historic bridge. Installing the pump was a cooperative effort between the Idaho Department of Environmental Quality and Kootenai County Waterways Department. The pump extends down approximately 120 feet into the Rathdrum Prairie Aquafer and delivers clean, fresh, cold water to trail users. The aquafer serves more than 370,000 residents in Kootenai County and Spokane County.

Historic Corbin Canal (Corbin Ditch)

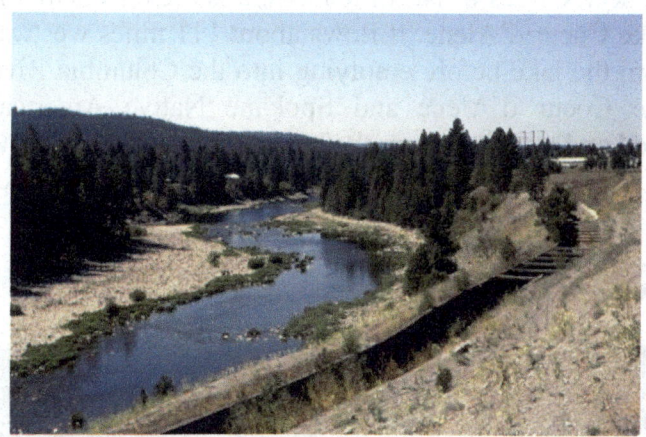

Photo by Doug Eastwood

Constructed in the late 1800's, this canal was an engineering marvel that carried water to the Spokane Valley and parts of the Rathdrum Prairie. It is credited with the expansion of agriculture and improved property values by irrigating an otherwise arid area. Part of the structure of the canal is still visible from the Centennial Trail. There is a trail head parking lot just west of Spokane Street on Fourth Street in Post Falls. The site of the Corbin Ditch is about 1/10 of a mile west of the parking lot along the Centennial Trail. You will be overlooking the Spokane River at this point. Between the Spokane River, and where you will be standing are the remnants of the Corbin Ditch that carried water westward into the Spokane Valley.

Spokane River: The Spokane River meanders through the scenic trees of North Idaho and is the only outlet for Lake Coeur d'Alene. It flows about 111 miles westward from the lake before emptying into the Columbia River. The Coeur d'Alene and Spokane Native Americans lived and traveled along the banks of this river. The river can be observed from many places along the trail route

Avista Island High Bridge

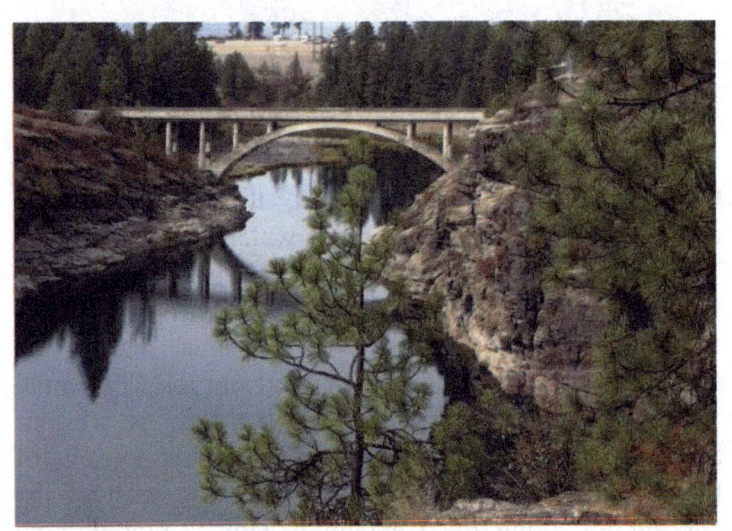

Photo by P.F. Parks Dept.

This is used as an access bridge for Avista Utilities to reach their hydroelectric operation. The bridge is viewable along the trail route and from Falls Park (west of Spokane St. and 4th) in the City of Post Falls. It spans over the Spokane River just north of the dam outlet.

Avista Dam at Falls Park

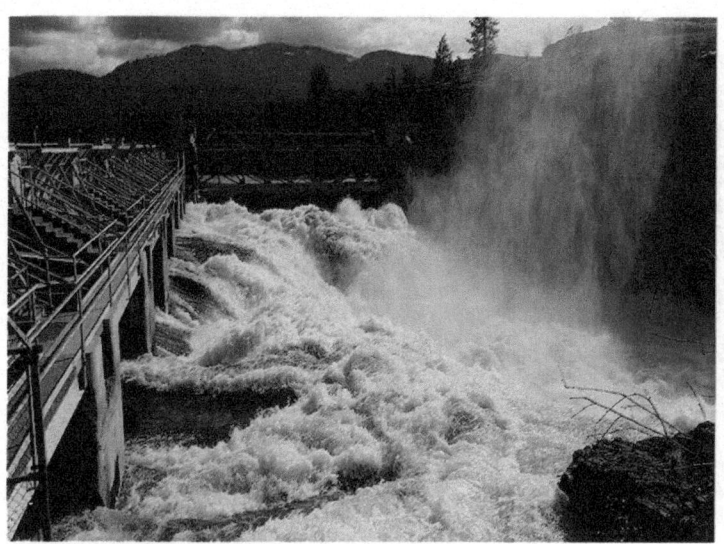

Photo by Doug Eastwood

There is a lot of history at this site. Frederick Post harnessed the water power as far back as the 1870's to power a lumber mill. In 1902 the mill burned down and was rebuilt in 1905. Washington Water Power (now Avista Utilities) bought the site with plans to develop a hydro-electric plant. Spring is the best time to see the dam as it is fully opened and the nearly 40-foot waterfall roars with mist shooting upwards of 100 feet. Falls Park is the best place to access these views. It is immediately off of the Centennial Trail on Fourth Street. In the winter time you can see natures beauty in the form of ice on the rocks beyond the dam outlet. Falls Park has parking, restrooms, picnic tables and walking paths leading to incredible view platforms of the dam and the river. Notice the mist rising from the water.

Treaty Rock

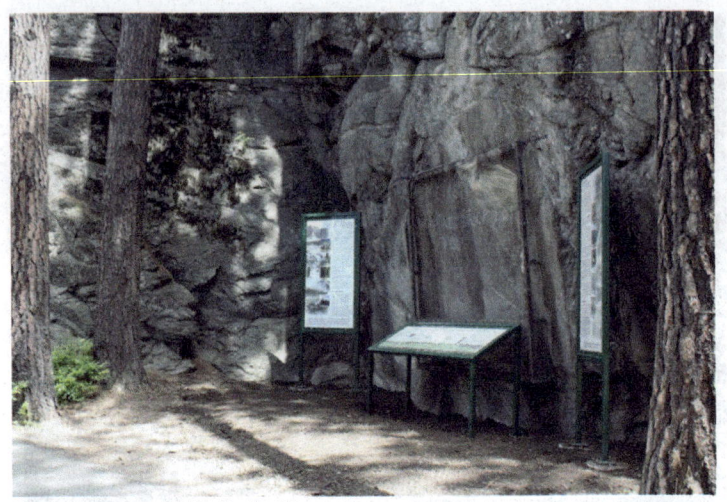

Photo by Post Falls Parks Dept.

This historic site was named Treaty Rock not because of an actual treaty, but because of an agreement between Frederick Post and Chief Seltice. Frederick Post needed to acquire nearly 200 acres of Spokane River property from the Chief. He needed the land for a lumber mill and this site is where the agreement took place. Chief Seltice required that his people be supplied with lumber material as part of the deal. The agreement was painted on a rock which has become known as Treaty Rock. The Treaty Rock site can be accessed from the Fourth Street Centennial Trail head parking lot.

Post Falls Museum at Fourth and Spokane Streets: The former building housing the Post Falls Parks and Recreation Department is now the Post Falls Museum. This nearly century old historic building is the perfect home for the city's museum. It is located on the NE corner of Spokane Street and 4th Street. The Centennial Trail passes just south of this location. Stop in and see the history of the City of Post Falls.

Post Falls Visitors Center: The visitor's center is located on Fourth Street just east of the museum. Information on the Post Falls area, local events, things to do, places to stay, shopping and services can all be found in this location.

Atlas Park: This new park being built by the City of Coeur d'Alene will be completed in 2020/2021. Atlas Park is located just south of Seltice Way on Atlas Road and it intersects the Centennial Trail and the Prairie Trail along the Spokane River. Parking, restrooms and other park amenities will be available.

Riverstone Park: Approaching Riverstone Park, and continuing throughout the next 11 miles, a variety of artwork, including murals, sculptures, chain saw carvings and other original creations will be noticeably visible. Each piece of artwork has a plaque identifying the work and the name of the artist. This Park is just about midway along the 23-mile Centennial Trail corridor. It hosts a man-made lake encircled by a paved pedestrian path. Water features and several pieces of art work are located in Riverstone Park. Free concerts are offered every Thursday night throughout the summer, compliments of the CDA Chamber of Commerce. Parking and restrooms are also available.

Kate and her Dogs – First Centennial Trail Sculpture

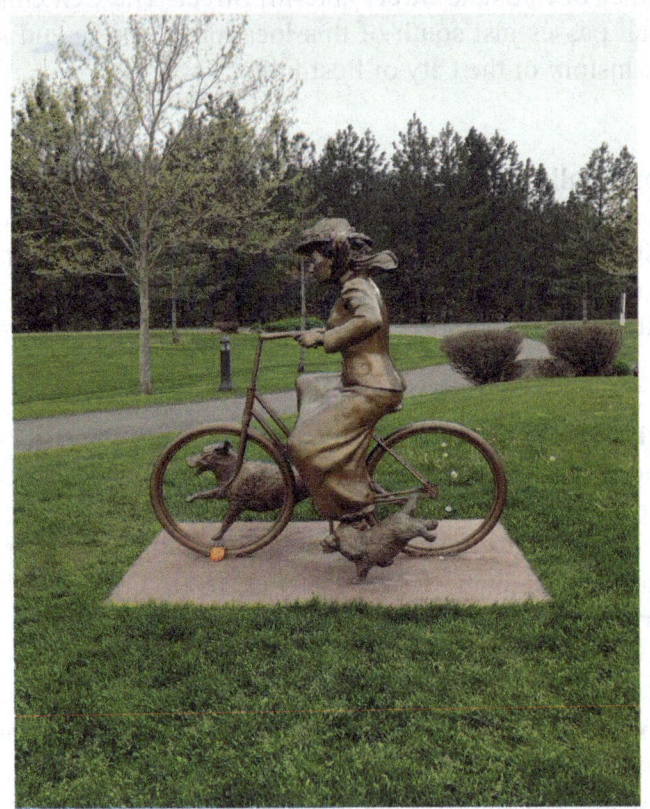

Photo by Doug Eastwood

One of the very first art sculptures is of a lady on a bike with her dogs running along-side. This artwork is close to the trail in Riverstone Park. This was a gift from the North Idaho Centennial Trail Foundation to the City of Coeur d'Alene in 2005.

North Idaho College: The college is located on one of the most beautiful sites in Idaho, along the Spokane River where it intersects with Lake Coeur d'Alene. The Centennial Trail travels along the river side of the college, and as you look north onto the campus you will be in awe of its setting and scenery. This is also the site of Fort Sherman, named for General William T. Sherman of the Civil War fame. As forts go, this one was not in operation very long, about 20 years. The soldiers from the fort were sent into the Spanish-American War. After the war, the fort was abandoned. Remnants of the fort are still on the college campus grounds including officers' quarters.

Historic Coeur d'Alene City Park 1880's (Originally, Blackwell Park): This is Coeur d'Alene's oldest park. Frederick Blackwell, a timber and transportation entrepreneur worked out an agreement with the federal government to develop the site into a park. This was a stopping place for one of his railroads and the park added to the adventure of traveling to Coeur d'Alene. The city eventually took responsibility for the park land. It is not clear when the name changed from Blackwell Park to Coeur d'Alene City Park. The Park sits on the north shore of Lake Coeur d'Alene and on the edge of the downtown area. It remains one of the most popular park sites in Idaho, averaging upwards of 2,000 to 3,000 visitors every day in the summer months. A free summer concert can be enjoyed every Sunday afternoon at the Rotary Lakeside Bandshell. The Centennial Trail passes through this historic park where you can find an abundance of art work. Jon Mueller, the design architect of the Centennial Trail wrote a book: *Private Park*

THE TRAIL THAT ALMOST WASN'T

Public Park – A Story of Coeur d'Alene and its First Park

Fort Sherman Playground

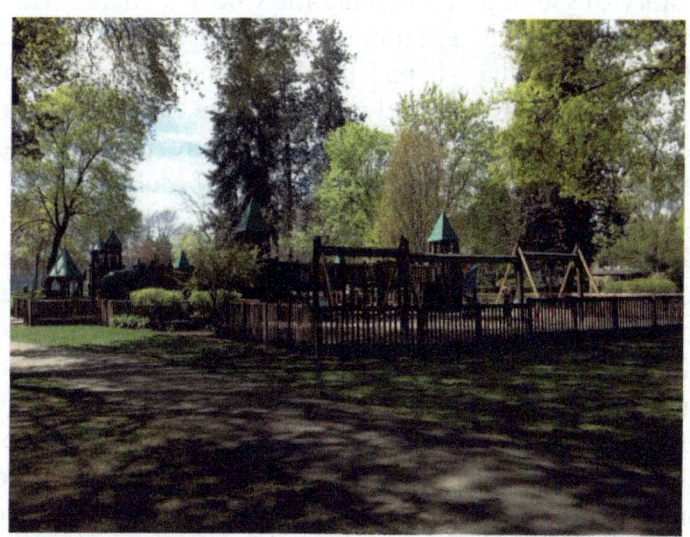

Photo by CDA Parks Dept

Located in the Coeur d'Alene City Park, the nearly ½ acre playground was introduced as an idea by Bliss Bignall, a local attorney and member of the Panhandle Kiwanis Club. The playground was a design-build project managed by Leathers and Associates from Ithaca, New York, an architectural firm that found a niche designing playgrounds throughout the country. The playground was built in 5 days with the help of 2,000 volunteers and more than $250,000 in donations of materials, tools and food to feed the volunteers. Nearly 1,700 engraved pickets surrounding the playground were sold to help raise funds for the project. The playground was completed in May of 1997. Caution: taking your kids into this playground may bring the kid out in you.

North Idaho Museum: The museum depicts the rich history of the region including the Coeur d'Alene Tribe, sawmills, logging, agriculture, railroads, steamboats and all the things that shaped the local and regional area. The museum is currently located on Sherman Ave. adjacent to the CDA City Park. There are plans to relocate the museum on the south side of McEuen Park.

Human Rights Education Institute: The HREI was formed in 1981 when the Kootenai County Task Force on Human Relations was founded by a diverse group of citizens as a response against the harassment and criminal activities of the Aryan Nations. This historic brick building was originally built and used by Spokane-Coeur d'Alene Electric Railroad. The HREI is located on the corner of Sherman Ave. and Fort Ground Drive adjacent to the CDA City Park.

Lake Coeur d'Alene: This is one of the most incredible features for a trail system anywhere in the country. The beauty of the lake coupled with the scenery of the Spokane River elevates the trail experience.

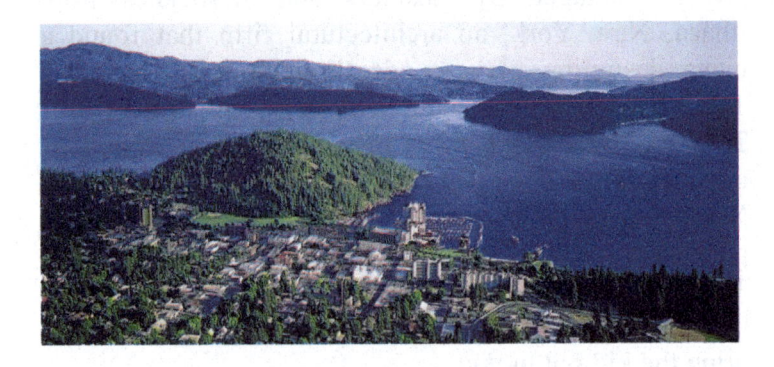

Your first encounter with the lake occurs as you leave the North Idaho College area towards the Coeur d'Alene

City Park. This natural lake, controlled by a dam was named after the Coeur d'Alene tribe, who were given their name by French explorers. The lake scenery along the final five miles of the trail is unparalleled.

Independence Point: The former site of Playland Pier. The pier burned down in 1974 and the waterfront park was built to commemorate our nations independence. The Park opened in 1976. Independence Point is immediately east of the Coeur d'Alene City Park. Lake cruises, seaplane rides, paddle boards and canoes are available at the Independence Point Commercial Docks.

Centennial Trail Monument

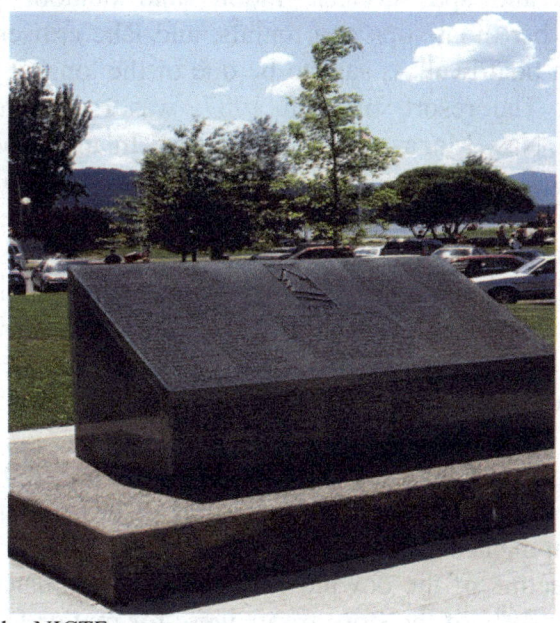

Photo by NICTF

This monument signifies the result of the first major fund raiser for the Centennial Trail in 1988-1989. This monument is located in the Independence Point Parking Lot adjacent to the Centennial Trail. Individuals and businesses can have their names engraved on the monument for $150.00. There are approximately 200 of the 2,500 spaces still available.

Coeur d'Alene Convention and Visitors Bureau: Located directly across the street from Independence Point. The visitor's bureau offers information on sight-seeing activities, places to visit, and just about anything else related to the Coeur d'Alene area.

Coeur d'Alene Resort: This world-famous resort includes several restaurants and lounges, boutiques, shuttle and spa services, indoor and outdoor pools, coffee bar, boat slips and rentals, and lake cruises. The marina boardwalk is said to be one of the longest in the world. The resort, built in 1987, was recognized by Conte Nas Magazine as the 'Best Inland Hotel in America'. Thousands of red geraniums are planted throughout the grounds every spring. Late November, the day after Thanksgiving, The Resort flips a switch and displays one of the most spectacular Christmas Light shows in the country. An added feature is a lake cruise to the 'North Pole' leaving from the resort docks all through the holiday season.

Downtown Coeur d'Alene: In the early 1980's the downtown area witnessed an exodus of businesses. The development of indoor shopping malls played a role in this decline of the downtown area. It is estimated that 30% to 40% of the store fronts were for rent or for sale. Downtown rallied with help from the City of Coeur d'Alene and established a 'Main Street USA' theme. By the late 1980's, new streets, lighting, sidewalks, utilities and perseverance by the store owners turned the area into one of the most vibrant downtowns in all of Idaho.

McEuen Park: This 20-acre waterfront park was for years a seasonal use ball field complex. The seasonal use of this prime piece of waterfront real estate benefited a relatively small percentage of city residents. A new park design was introduced and developed in 2013-2014. Its current popularity and number of visitors now mirror that of the historic Coeur d'Alene City Park. It is host to numerous outdoor activities throughout the summer. Take a leisurely stroll around and through this park to appreciate all the amenities it has to offer. The Centennial Trail meanders through this park.

Tubbs Hill: A 120-acre natural park area located on the south side of McEuen Park and bordered by Lake Coeur d'Alene on the west, south and east. There is a two-mile hiking trail around the perimeter of the hill. Bikes are prohibited on Tubbs Hill to ensure its preservation and for safety purposes. An interpretive brochure is available at the CDA Parks office located at the east end of McEuen Park in city hall. The main entrance to Tubbs Hill is located at the southwest corner of McEuen Park. A memorial rock at the entrance to Tubbs Hill recognizes Scott Reed and Art Manley who fought diligently throughout the 1960's and 1970's to have the city acquire this hill and preserve it for the people forever. Scott Reed authored a book on this priceless land titled; *Tubbs Hill, A City Treasure*.

Mudgy and Millie

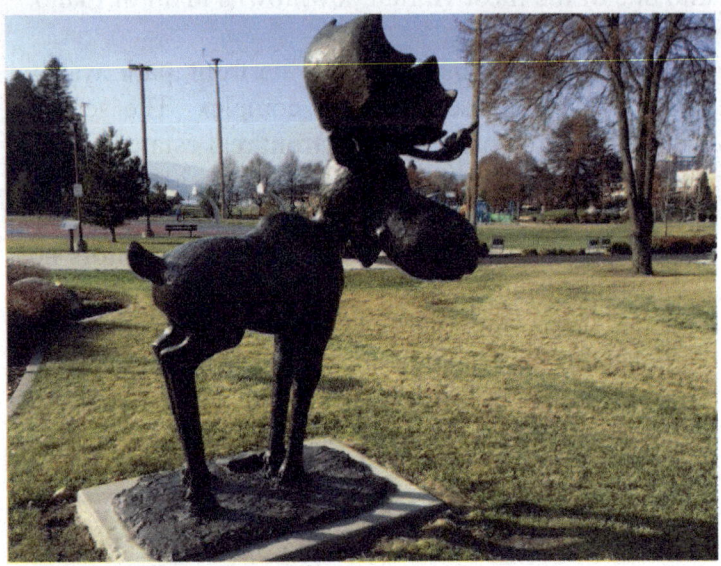

Photo by Doug Eastwood

Mudgy and Millie, authored and created by Susan Nipp, is the story of two friends, a moose and a mouse who travel together through the City of Coeur d'Alene. Their trek begins at the Coeur d'Alene Public Library and meanders through McEuen Park, Downtown Coeur d'Alene, Independence Point and finishes at the Coeur d'Alene City Park next to Fort Sherman Playground. *Mudgy and Millie* is an interactive adventure that encourages kids (and adults) to walk the trail to each of the designated sites, identified by near life size sculptures of the moose and mouse. It has been rumored that Mudgy and Millie have been spotted as far away as Australia and Costa Rica.

Coeur d'Alene Resort Golf Course (Former site of the Rutledge Mill): This nearly 140-acre lumber mill site was acquired by CDA Resort owner, Duane Hagadone, and converted to a world-renowned lake side golf course. The golf course is home to the iconic floating green as well as a restaurant and pro shop. The Hagadone Event Center was recently added which is host to public and private events all year around.

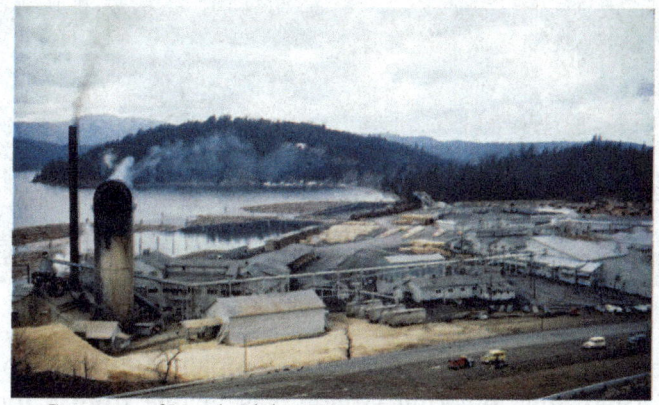

Photo Courtesy of North Idaho Museum
Rutledge Mill – Potlatch – 1950's

Lake Steamers Historic Site: This viewpoint is located along the Centennial Trail about two miles east of Coeur d'Alene. Steamers were large boats powered by steam engines and often propelled by paddle wheels. The U.S. Army used steamers to haul goods to Fort Sherman in Coeur d'Alene. Later, the steamers would haul ore, freight and passengers across Lake Coeur d'Alene. Steamers were common on the lake in the 1880's.

Veterans Memorial Bridge

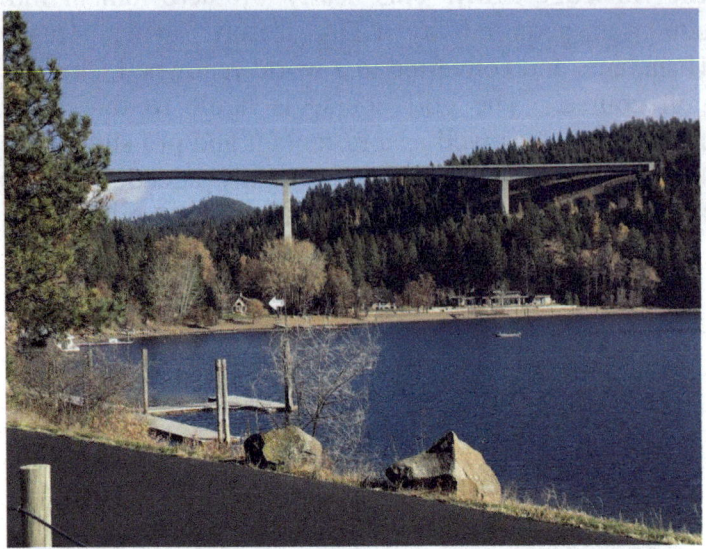

Photo by Doug Eastwood

Veterans Memorial Bridge was completed in September of 1990, this towering structure is visible from a long distance. Traveling along the Centennial Trail, eastward, it looms in the distance once you pass the Lake Steamers Historic Site. This bridge is 300 feet tall, 1,720 feet long and 83 feet wide. Interstate 90 used to be where the Centennial Trail is today. The Veterans Memorial Bridge was part of the I-90 relocation project.

Historic Beacon Point: Used for lake navigation and located about 4 miles east of Coeur d'Alene, the Centennial Trail encounters Beacon Point. This natural rock land mass extends into the lake and was once used as a navigation warning for big boats nearing the rock outcropping. There are pathways around the rock outcropping with viewpoints of the lake.

1990 Slide Area; Two dozers can be found at the bottom of lake. This is the site where part of I-90 slid into the lake during the I-90 relocation project.

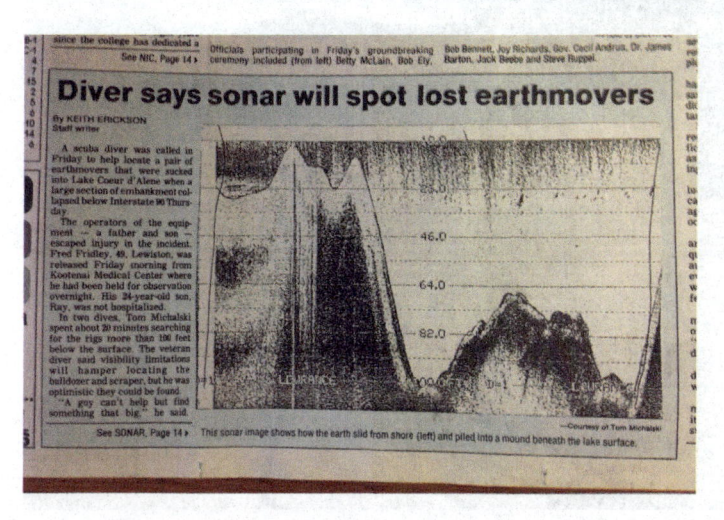

CDA Press May 19, 1990

This incident led to law suits being filed against the Idaho Transportation Department which ultimately led to the development of the Centennial Trail along the lake shoreline. This was done in mitigation of the damage to the lake and fish spawning areas. The site of the slide where the earth moving equipment went into the lake is between the boat launch and Higgins Point, or about 300 feet to the right of the photo below.

Circa 1900 Photographer Sculpture

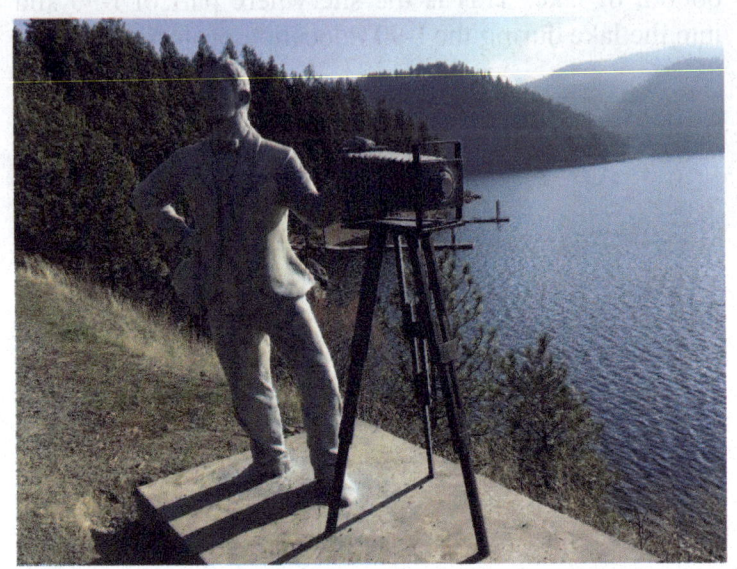

Photo by IDPR

This sculpture is located on the final few hundred feet of the Centennial Trail leading up to Higgins Point. The sculpture is that of a photographer and his camera mounted on a tri-pod. The era of his clothing and camera is said to be that of the early 1900's. Migratory birds were probably flocking to this area more than 100 years ago and perhaps the photographer was there to capture them in flight. Or maybe he was capturing some of the incredible scenery of the lake, mountains and the sunset.

Bald Eagle Migration Viewing Area: Higgins Point and surrounding areas are well known for attracting Eagle watchers. Beautiful and graceful, the eagles can be seen swooping down on the lake and pulling out Kokanee Salmon with their powerful talons. Other bird's native to the area are a bit nervous when the big birds return every fall.

Public Parking Locations:
- Southwest corner of Spokane Bridge Street and Appleway on the Washington side of the trail
- Treaty Rock in Post Falls, also known as the 4th Street Trail Head Parking
- Falls Park in Post Falls
- Frontier Ice Arena on Seltice Way in CDA, compliments of Ignite CDA
- Trail Head parking at northwest corner of Northwest Boulevard and Seltice Way
- Riverstone Park
- Memorial Field
- CDA City Park
- McEuen Park
- There are five parking lots along CDA Lake Drive to Higgins Point.
- Public streets anywhere parking is permitted along the trail route.

Photos on back and front covers are courtesy of Jon Jonkers and Doug Eastwood

THE TRAIL THAT ALMOST WASN'T

Map and QRC Code provided by Monte McCully

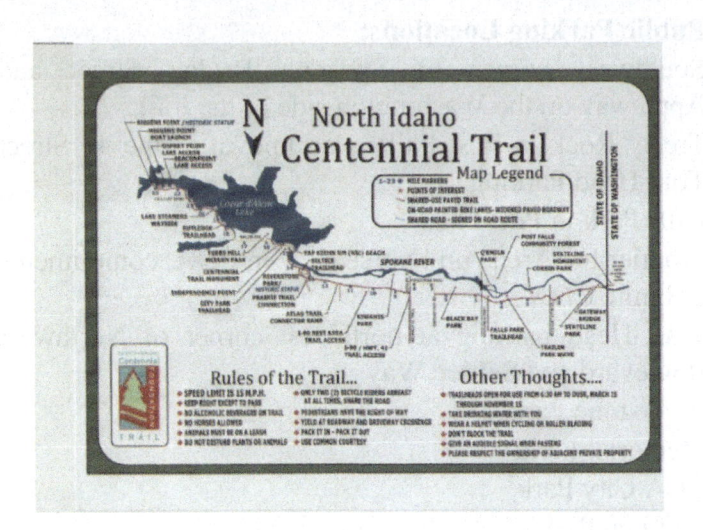

e

NORTH IDAHO CENTENNIAL TRAIL MAP
Includes the Spokane Centennial Trail
62 Miles of Urban Trail
From Higgins Point to Spokane

QRC – Use Your Cell Phone
To download the map

NORTH IDAHO CENTENNIAL TRAIL

REFERENCES & NOTES

Abandoned Railroads, Title 49, Chapter 10, Code of Federal Regulations

American Forest Magazine 2015. Greenways & Rambling - Ideas for Healthier Cities

American Journal of Cardiology 2018

Brooks, J. Rebecca 2018 *The Industrial Revolution in America*

Burlington Northern Railroad History. Wikipedia
    Coeur d'Alene Parks Department
    Coeur d'Alene Press; 1987 – 1992
    Coeur d'Alene Public Library

ConservationTools.org: Economic Benefits of trails 2015 – 2019

Crompton, L. John 2004 *The Proximate Principle* in cooperation with the National Recreation and Parks Association

Economic Benefits of Trails: American Trails Magazine 2011, 2014, 2017

Frontiers in Neuroscience 2018

Galic, Bohana 2019 www.livstrong.com *Psychology Today*

Health Benefits of a Pedestrian-Bicycle Trail: National Recreation and Parks Association 2016

Houda, Kegan 2005 The Corbin Ditch. Spokane Historical

Idaho Department of Lands

Idaho Transportation Department

Kanter, Rosabeth Moss 2012 *Change Management.* Ten Reasons People Resist Change

Kootenai County Parks & Waterways

Kootenai County Prosecuting Attorney Seltice Way Opinion 1989

Peterson, Steven – Research Economist 2019 The *Economic Impact of the North Idaho Centennial Trail*

Post Falls Parks & Recreation

Rails with Trails: Lessons Learned, Federal Highway Administration, June 2017

Robert Dellwo Memorandum to IDFG 1987

Spokesman Review; 1987-1990

Ward, Thomas PHD 2017 *Psychology Today*

www.AmericanTrails.com 2016
    www.burkegilmantrail Friends of the Burke-Gilman Trail

www.burlingtonnorthernrailroad 2016

www.railstotrailsconservancy 2011 History of Rail-Trails. RTC Timeline. History and Evolution

Acknowledgements

I have been encouraged for years to document the history of the North Idaho Centennial Trail. My involvement with the trail dates back to 1986 when the idea was first introduced. I was unaware, at that time, that documenting the trail history would result in the creation of this book.

Many people, too numerous to mention, have been instrumental in turning this vision into a reality. I want to thank those who were there with me from the very beginning of the trail's inception and contributed to the information provided in this book: Bob Mcdonald, Evalyn Adams, Randy Haddock, and Lance Bridges. Many thanks as well to Dave Fair, Steve McCrae, Bob Nelson, Kent Helmer, Sandy Emerson, and the late Scott Reed for their support during the trail development. I want to recognize Jon Mueller for his work on the trail design and providing me access to his notes and photos, and thanks to the North Idaho Centennial Trail Board of Directors.

I am grateful to the City of Coeur d'Alene for allowing me to pursue the vision and development of this legacy trail during my many years employed by the city. Thanks to the Coeur d'Alene Public Library for their volumes of chronological newspaper articles and the North Idaho Museum for giving me access to their photo files.

I also want to thank author, Jack Castle, for advice helping me through the writing maze and publishing methodology. Thanks to Suzanne Holland for her incredible editing skills.

Finally, I want to thank my wife Dee, my daughters Alicia and Valerie, and my niece Carly Davis.

About the Author

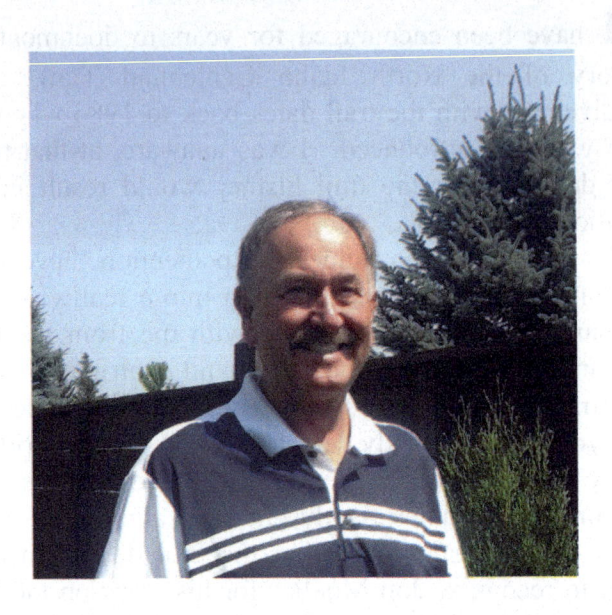

Doug Eastwood began his career with the County of Los Angeles, Parks and Recreation Department in 1972. He was promoted to park administration at a 2,000-acre site that boasted of a man-made lake called Puddingstone, boat launch, docks, a golf course, equestrian trails, massive group and family picnic areas and a sand bottom outdoor pool. During his time with L.A. County, he pursued a degree in Landscape Construction at Mt. San Antonio College. He also had the opportunity to study under one of the top botanists in the world; Dr. H. Hamilton Williams III at L.A. Trade Technical College.

In 1978, before completing his education, he relocated with his wife and infant daughter to North Idaho. He completed his education, obtaining two bachelor degrees from Lewis and Clark State College.

For the next 35 years he worked for, and directed, the City of Coeur d'Alene Parks Department, retiring in 2013. During that time, he grew the city's park system from five parks to 32 parks including miles of pedestrian and bicycle paths and the North Idaho Centennial Trail.

He served as president of the Idaho Recreation and Parks Association and member of the National Parks and Recreation Association. He was a member of the Kiwanis Panhandle Club where he served as president and Lt. Governor of Kiwanis for the Idaho Panhandle. During his time with Kiwanis, the club spearheaded the development of Fort Sherman Playground in the Coeur d'Alene City Park.

Currently Doug is on the board of directors with the North Idaho Centennial Trail Foundation and a board member for the Idaho Department of Parks and Recreation.

Doug assisted with the formation of the Tubbs Hill Foundation and the North Idaho Centennial Trail Foundation. He introduced the creation of the Panhandle Parks Foundation.

Throughout most of his career, Doug enjoyed long-distance bicycling, and now his retirement has allowed him to expand his interests. Today he enjoys wood working, bowling, ATV riding, snowshoeing, traveling and volunteer work. He also enjoys speaking to groups, being entertained by his dogs and spending time with his grand-daughters.

Made in the USA
Columbia, SC
09 February 2025